COVID-19 Pandemic

Critically analyzing the specific security threat posed by COVID-19 to global society, the contributors to this book offer a comprehensive and critical examination of global challenges and responses while suggesting more balanced and nuanced approaches to handling these security impacts.

The COVID-19 pandemic brought about a huge challenge to health security across the globe. Several countries were pushed into lockdown repeatedly to prevent the spread of infection. The global economy has seen a major slowdown and disruption of supply chains around the world. There have also been major implications from changes to traditional security systems as well as diverse societal change even down to aspects of daily life. The chapters in this book show that progressive initiatives have expended a mixture of soft and hard response strategies that include understanding, containing, fighting, and preventing COVID-19. They look at major sectors including defense, trade, health, and bioterrorism among others. In doing so, they highlight the best practices used around the world to minimize the threat posed by COVID-19's impact.

A vital resource for security studies scholars and policymakers.

Rohan Kumar Gunaratna is Professor of Security Studies at the S. Rajaratnam School of International Studies, Nanyang Technology University, and Founder of International Centre for Political Violence and Terrorism Research, Singapore. He received his Masters from the University of Notre Dame in the United States where he was a Hesburgh Scholar and his doctorate from the University of St Andrews in the United Kingdom where he was a British Chevening Scholar. A former Senior Fellow at the Combating Terrorism Centre at the United States Military Academy at West Point and the Fletcher School of Law and Diplomacy, Gunaratna was Visiting Fellow at the Washington Institute for Near East Policy. The author of "Inside al Qaeda: Global Network of Terror" (University of Columbia Press), Gunaratna, edited the Insurgency and Terrorism Series of the Imperial College Press, London. A trainer for national security agencies, law enforcement authorities, and military counterterrorism units, he interviewed terrorists and insurgents in Afghanistan, Pakistan, Iraq, Yemen, Libya, Saudi Arabia, and other conflict zones. For advancing international security cooperation, Gunaratna received the Major General Ralph H. Van Deman Award.

Mohd Mizan Aslam is Professor of Strategic Studies at the Universiti Malaysia Perlis (UniMAP), and founder and first director of Malaysian Research Institute of Strategic Studies (MyRISS). Mizan was conferred Honorary Major by Malaysian Armed Forces in 2016 due to his contribution in security and CVE initiatives. He is also a national expert panel in rehabilitation programs to terrorist inmates nationwide. He is a writer for numerous books, conference papers, journals, proceedings, newspapers, magazines, keynote speakers, and TV and news columnists. Mizan actively involves in fellowship abroad as Executive Council of Benevolent Fund for Outstanding Students (BFOS), Hadramowt, Govt of Yemen, and Executive Advisor QATAR Guest Centre, Doha Qatar. Mizan held a position as Adjunct Professor at School of Arts & Humanities, Universitas Ubudiyah Indonesia (UUI), Acheh, Indonesia. Mizan also appointed as Visiting Professor at the Centre for Civilization & Peace Study, Ibnu Haldun University, Beheksehir, Istanbul, Turkey in 2017. Mizan involved in developing a National Action Plan on CVE with Home Ministry of Malaysia and also appointed as Senior Fellow at Islamic and Strategic Studies Institute (ISSI-CONCAVE).

Routledge Studies in the Politics of Disorder
and Instability

COVID-19 Pandemic

The Threat and Response

Edited by Rohan Kumar Gunaratna
and Mohd Mizan Aslam

Routledge
Taylor & Francis Group

LONDON AND NEW YORK

First published 2022
by Routledge
2 Park Square, Milton Park, Abingdon, Oxon OX14 4RN

and by Routledge
605 Third Avenue, New York, NY 10158

*Routledge is an imprint of the Taylor & Francis Group,
an Informa business*

British Library Cataloguing-in-Publication Data
A catalogue record for this book is available from the British Library

Library of Congress Cataloguing-in-Publication Data
A catalog record has been requested for this book

ISBN: 9781032054049 (hbk)
ISBN: 9781032054063 (pbk)
ISBN: 9781003197416 (ebk)

DOI: 10.4324/9781003197416

Typeset in Galliard
by KnowledgeWorks Global Ltd.

We are in this together - and we will get through this, together.

Antonio Guterres, UN Secretary – 2020.

Contents

Figures

Tables

Contributors

Shane Britten has worked in homeland security and counterterrorism for more than 15 years, including as an intelligence officer with the Australian Government. He has provided intelligence capability building around the world, including throughout Southeast Asia, the Middle East, and Africa. Since leaving government in 2014, Mr Britten has worked as the CEO of a multi-national software business and the Head of National Security and Intelligence for an Australian information security business. He lectures at universities on building homeland security capability and continues to be a key advisor for governments in Southeast Asia on terrorism issues. He has a Bachelor of Biotechnology (Microbiology and Genetic Engineering) with Honours from the University of Queensland.

Richard J. Chasdi is an adjunct assistant professor at the Center for Peace and Conflict Studies at Wayne State University and an adjunct associate professor in the Department of Political Science at the University of Windsor. His three books include "Counterterror Offensives for the Ghost War World: The Rudiments of Counterterrorism Policy" (Lexington Books, 2010), "Tapestry of Terror: A Portrait of Middle East Terrorism, 1994–1999" (Lexington Books, 2002), and "Serenade of Suffering: A Portrait of Middle East Terrorism 1968–1993" (Lexington Books, 1999 – CHOICE magazine "Outstanding Academic Title" 2000). Dr Chasdi has written academic articles and book chapters and is a member of the Editorial Board of Perspectives on *Terrorism: A Journal of the Terrorism Research Initiative*, where he writes a monthly "Research Note." He also serves on the International Advisory Board of Terrorism: An Electronic Journal & Knowledge Base. In addition, he is an adjunct faculty member at Walsh College.

Sophie Drake is a graduate of Oxford University and the London School of Economics and Politics Science. With a BA in Theology and an MSc in Social Anthropology, Sophie has specialized in Islamic theology and Political Islam. Sophie has worked for a number of international think tanks and NGOs in the areas of international relations, globalization, and development. Her expertise lies in human security, with a focus on counterterrorism and countering violent extremism.

Rusdi Omar is the Dean of Ghazali Shafie Graduate School of Government (GSGSG) at College of Law, Government and International Studies (COL-GIS) Universiti Utara Malaysia (UUM). He received his PhD in Politics and International Studies from Adelaide University, Australia, and Master of Law in International Relations from Hitotsubashi University, Japan. Dr Rusdi also holds a Bachelor of Degree in Economics (Hons) from Universiti Malaya, Malaysia. He teaches both undergraduate and post-graduate courses, which include International Relations, Foreign Policy Analysis, Malaysian Foreign Policy, Diplomacy, Politics of Developed and Developing Countries, and East Asian Politics. His primary research interests include International Relations, Malaysian Politics, Malaysia–Singapore Relations, Southeast Asian/East Asian Politics, Political Leadership, and Foreign Policy Analysis. Apart from that, Dr Rusdi has published many articles in international and national refereed journals include with the status of Scopus/ISI indexed and also in conference proceedings. He has published several books and book chapters. Regarding on student supervision, he has supervised many undergraduate and post-graduate students in the areas of his expertise. It is also important to note that he also regularly sought after and featured in the national mass media for his commentaries on various political and security issues in Malaysia and Singapore.

Nihal Pitigala is an Economist with over 25 years of experience in trade and development with international organizations such as the World Bank, USAID, and the EU. He specializes in providing policy-relevant research and has worked in 25 countries across Asia, Sub-Saharan Africa, and the Middle East. He has published several peer-reviewed articles on trade integration, export competitiveness, and regional and global value chains and has taught trade policy courses to academia and government officials. At the World Bank, he has supported both research and operational work. He also assisted in the development of the World Bank Group Trade Strategy that was launched in 2011. He holds a PhD in Economics from the University of Sussex.

Animesh Roul is the Executive Director of New Delhi-based policy research group Society for the Study of Peace and Conflict. He specializes in counterterrorism, radical Islam, religious eschatology, and issues related to armed conflict and insurgencies in South Asia. Roul has written extensively on these subject areas in journals and policy magazines including the CTC Sentinel, Jane's Intelligence Review, and CBW Magazine, among others. He has been associated with the Jamestown Foundation (Washington DC) since 2005 as a South Asia Counterterrorism analyst and regularly contributes to the Foundation's landmark publications "Terrorism Monitor" and "Militant Leadership Monitors." He co-authored a book on India's indigenous terror group, "Indian Mujahideen: Computational Analysis and Public Policy" (Springer, New York, 2013). His latest paper, "Coronavirus as God's Soldier: Assessing the Divine Retribution Narrative of Jihadi Organisations" has been published in an edited book "COVID-19: Analysing the Threat" (Pentagon Press, New Delhi, 2020). Presently he is coediting a book titled "The Handbook of Terrorist and Insurgent Groups: Tactics, Strategies, and Characteristics" (CRC Press.).

Chandra Nilanga Samarasinghe MA, MB, BS. Free Lance Researcher in Health Economics and Health Policies. Chandra is a former researcher at the Department of Health Sciences and Medicine, University of Luzern, Switzerland. He is also former Chair Person of the National Dangerous Drugs (Narcotics) Control Board and Precursor Chemicals Control Authority of Sri Lanka. He was the Head of the Department of Infection Control and Health Education of NHRD, Sri Lanka Obstetrician and Gynecologist at NCTH, Sri Lanka, and Forensic Pathologist at NCTH, Sri Lanka. Chandra obtained Masters in Health Sciences with double majors in Health Economics and Health Policies from the University of Luzern, Switzerland. He also obtained Bachelor in Medicine and Bachelor in Surgery with second class Honor from the Faculty of Medicine, University of Kelaniya, Sri Lanka. Chandra's involved in International Engagements such as the founding member of South Asian Regional Council against Trans Nations Organized Crimes, New Delhi, 2015, resource Person of the Gulf Summit for International Drugs Trafficking, Doha, Qatar, 2015, focal point of the United Nations Office of Drugs and Crimes 2015, resource Person at World Hepatitis Day Seminar, Colombo, Sri Lanka, 2015, special training on Drugs Control at Yunnan Police Academy, Yunnan, Kunming, China, member of Swiss representation at the workshop for Public Health Disaster Management Program at Sichuan University, Chengdu, China 2019. Currently, he is the Health Communicator, Public Speaker and Journalist in Social and Civil Activist.

Rasitha Wickramsinghe has over 20 years of client-facing experience in European and Asian markets. He joined Stax in February 2015 and leads the Business Development team for APAC region. He is responsible for initiating new client engagements, advising existing clients, and taking the Stax brand to new geographies. At Stax, Rasitha has led multiple engagements with local and international clients across diverse sectors such as financial services, retail, hospitality, education, and industrial manufacturing. Local clients he advises include diversified conglomerates, listed companies, family owned businesses, and startups. Prior to joining Stax, Rasitha was a Business Development Director at a technology subsidiary of MAS Holdings. Rasitha started his career in the telecommunications industry working as a consultant for Nokia and then Telefonica-O2 in the UK. He managed pan European client engagements with leading telcos such as Vodafone Group, Orange Group, Telefonica Group, and Hutchinson 3G. Rasitha holds a PhD from Sheffield Hallam University, Sheffield, UK. He also holds an MBA from Warwick Business School, UK, and honors degree in Electrical & Electronic Engineering from South Bank University, London.

Thomas Wuchte joined the International Institute for Justice and the Rule of Law (IIJ) as Executive Director from his position as the Head on Anti-Terrorism Issues in the Organization for Security and Co-operation in Europe (OSCE). He is a graduate of the United States Military Academy at West Point and received a post-graduate degree in International Relations from the University of Illinois. Before his duties at the IIJ and OSCE, Mr Wuchte received the US Department of State's Highest Award for Excellence in International Security Affairs for his efforts to work collaboratively with international partners.

Knocks Tapiwa Zengeni is a Visiting Senior Scholar and specialist on American Politics and International Security with the School of International Studies, College of Government, Law and International Studies, Universiti Utara Malaysia, Kedah, Malaysia. He received his PhD in International Studies (Politics) from the Universiti Utara Malaysia. He has also held teaching appointments at the University of Zimbabwe and Africa University (Zimbabwe). Dr Zengeni is a former senior government official in Zimbabwe. His research interests include comparative politics, media & politics, foreign policy analysis, international relations theory, and international security. He is the author of several book chapters and articles dealing with issues in Africa, Asia as well as globally. He is an Associate Editor of the African Journal of Defence and Security and co-author of a book entitled International Relations (Pearson, Singapore, 2014). Currently, he is working on a book on Malaysia–Singapore Relations and the Mahathir Factor.

Preface

The first edition of the COVID-19 response was envisioned to measure the formative phase of the pandemic raged the whole world in early 2020. In this book, we aimed to describe a variety of efforts that reflects the wide range of response currently being performed as COVID-19 threat & response. This volume provides a rich array of perspectives on the world's most serious challenges. Scholars, analysts, and practitioners from all around the world voice their outlooks through many unique lenses. This volume critically analyzes the specific threat posed by COVID-19 to the global society. It offers a comprehensive and critical examination of COVID-19 global responses and challenges, suggesting more balanced and nuanced approaches to handling the impact. Contributors include leading scholars in global security, economics, public health, ICT, bioterrorism, political issues, and religious conflict. These cross-continental experts include renowned world security analysts, as well as highly regarded ex-military officers, journalists, academics, medical practitioners, and overall outstanding commentators. The recent COVID-19 pandemic has brought about a huge challenge to health security across the globe. Several countries have been pushed into lockdown to prevent the spread of infection. The global economy has seen a major slowdown and disruption of supply chains around the world. There have also been major implications of change to traditional security systems as well as diverse societal change down to aspects of daily life. Complexity is the major issue in defining the best solution to COVID-19. However, this is the right time for us to come up with specific platforms to reassess needs and wants. Thus, this task has emerged as a major policy concern and has challenged states in their COVID-19 responses. The chapters in this volume have demonstrated that progressive initiatives have expended a milieu of soft and hard response strategies that include understanding, containing, fighting, and preventing COVID-19. It was supported with the best method to prevent panic and catastrophe. These have been represented in quick responses including quarantine, control order, closing borders, and social distancing, taken by countries in order to ensure the success of the war against this deadly virus. The choice of a framework for fighting COVID-19 is by no means straightforward. It is intricate and requires a deep study on an array of factors that will be positively responded to by the overall system. The volume's outcome was an understanding of the impact and threat

COVID-19 posed to the world's security and was intended to help governments and policymakers to revisit their whole of security-related policy and prevent their country from deteriorating into chaos resulting from COVID-19 or any pandemic threat in the future. The second edition of the COVID-19 response focuses on Asia will be published in 2022.

Acknowledgments

To defeat the global pandemic, the world has come together. Through this book, we have brought together scholars and practitioners working on facets of the COVID-19 pandemic. Their research focuses on the post-COVID-19 impact on global security around the world. Gunaratna and Mizan would like to thank the contributing authors for participating in an unprecedented project. We are indebted to the valuable suggestions by the reviewers. In Singapore, we would like to express our gratitude by thanking our research assistants, Clifford Gere and Glenda Tan of the S. Rajaratnam School of International Studies and Rochelle Teo of the Department of Psychology, the Nanyang Technology University (NTU), Singapore. Our special thanks go to Vanessa Lim Panes, Vlad Antonio, Sievalee Wijayawardhana, and Tristan Muralitharan for their research assistance.

We would also like to thank Kasiviswanathan Shanmugam, Minister of Home Affairs of Singapore, Tito Karnavian, Minister of Home Affairs of Indonesia, and Dato' Sri Ismail Sabri, the Defence and Security Minister of Malaysia, for their vision. Many in government, both past and present, especially the visionary leadership Mr Benny Lim led to creating a research culture in security studies. Similarly, in Malaysia, our deepest appreciation goes to Deputy Commissioner Datuk Ayob Khan Mydin Pitchay, Prof Dr Shahimi Moktar of UUM, Dr Fahad Alharby, Dr Sayed Ameer of NAUSS, and Prof Ir Ts Dr R Badlishah of UniMAP for fostered cooperation between the government, community organizations, and academia.

We thank the staff of the International Centre for Political Violence and Terrorism Research (ICPVTR) at NTU, Singapore, Universiti Malaysia Perlis (UniMAP) and Naif Arab University for Security Sciences (NAUSS), Riyadh, KSA, for their steadfast assistance in supporting research on national and international security threats and response during the pandemic.

Foreword

The COVID-19 pandemic matters to the whole world; while we can't predict exactly when or where the next outbreak will begin, we know one is coming just in a matter of time. Unprecedented tragedies in the modern world shocked every single country; it thereby appears that in managing such a threat, timely response is the key to success. Defense and security as a premier frontliner, maintain mission readiness, ensure public safety and support government-wide efforts in a wide range of areas by prompt and precise response to the threat of COVID-19. How we stop outbreaks from becoming widespread pandemics that threaten us all will be an indicator that ensures the sustainability of Malaysian citizens regardless of place and space.

COVID-19 takes hold in the world's most vulnerable areas, especially defense, education, health, food, religion, trade, and business activities. Countries with very little resources to stop the spread of infection before it reaches the shores will be left in bad situations. When a virus can travel from a secluded corner to major cities on all continents in less than two days, the threat to our national defense is greater than ever. Many challenges exist worldwide that increase the risk of pandemic and rapid spread, including:

- Act of terrorism
- Wake of digital acceleration
- Ability to travel
- Massive online trade and business
- Acts of bioterrorism
- Weaknesses of public health infrastructures
- Religious congregations and many more

The world must come forward together, taking steps to better detect, plan and respond to COVID-19; every single country has to develop a pre- and post-COVID-19 response system. This response will hold best practice that will allow better support in country's defense. A system planning and responsiveness, including the immediate need to analyze the current COVID-19 outbreak and the impact on every single aspect of the country also has to be developed.

With that, I congratulate Dr Mizan and Dr. Rohan on getting your timely book published! Precious few have had the nerve to write on the COVID-19 threat and response. You have written an excellent book that should raise lots of eyebrows. Of course, many of your chapters were done by hard-won researchers and practitioners in the matter. Nevertheless, both of you must have done a wheelbarrow-full of research on pandemic threat and response across disciplines. I admire your academic works. I guess this means we will be seeing more of you in the print media from now on. I say congratulations to both of you!

Dato' Sri Ismail Sabri Bin Yaakob
Deputy Prime Minister/
Senior Minister of Defence
Government of Malaysia

Introduction

Rohan Gunaratna and Mohd Mizan Aslam

The world is at the very early stages of a global pandemic that is likely to last for decades (Gunaratna, 2020). Unprecedented pandemic changes the life of modern society regardless of boundaries, religions, and social strata. Through a series of studies, both thematic and regional, we seek to understand the current and emerging threat and the global response. The COVID-19 pandemic that has threatened the world in particular, happened during the time when most countries were not ready Being in a comfortable and safe zone for a long period has made many countries feel too much at ease and unready to make earlier preparations to face this crisis (Aslam, 2020).

As we aspire to return to normalcy, the world we must individually and collectively build should be equitable and sustainable. It should neither be the pre- or the COVID World, but a world where we return to living a life where we break "cultural barriers, giving way to significant social momentum." The COVID-19 threat clearly shows the weakness of the global security management especially from aspects concerning defense, food safety, health, and other related sectors. The world is expected to be in a state of crisis if this pandemic continues for a long time. Even though it is obvious that COVID-19 has made a huge impact on the economy (Kalbana and Chan, 2020), the threat in terms of safety and defense aspects is very significant. Without economic growth, the security and defense industry of a country will be affected.

Developments in recent years have revealed that the world is facing global health challenges such as ZIKA, AIDS, SARS, EBOLA, and now COVID-19, which has become a major security issue for most countries around the world. This is because the issue of pandemic dominates every single country regardless of locality and size. In most cases, the main proponent which exacerbates the menace of pandemic is a lifestyle. Lifestyle is a strong force that could lead people to either act in a civilized or barbaric way of life. Dealing with the subject of pandemic is always an uphill task and difficult to overcome, given the experience of the larger world in previous catastrophes like Blackdeath, American-Polio, Yellow-Fever, and Great Plague of Marseille decades ago.

Currently, concerns have been raised as to how to deal with this unpleasant modern world problem known as COVID-19, which is a super spreader virus due to the impact of globalization. Realistically, the fight against the COVID-19 pandemic ends up with the loss of lives, time, and money in every single country in this world. These phenomena are detrimental to the lifestyle and have created a "new-normal" that lasts for decades. If governments around the world fail to tackle COVID-19 profoundly as it should, there could be a further deterioration of the problem with the possibilities of damaging the social and economic of the countries that will lead to great inflation, bankruptcy, and mass deaths.

The most effective remedy for curbing the menace of pandemic is the activation of a "new-normal" for as long as mankind continues to exist in this world. This has become imperative for every country in order to maintain socio-stability and economic prosperity. In this regard, several post-pandemic issues range from finance to digital, from west to east are being taken by every nation. The method and manner would depend on the "new-normal" and "strategies" for tackling health, food, technology, and defense security. The strategy was designed to cover the atmosphere or perimeter under threat. It covers both the preventive and corrective aspects of countering deadly viruses through new policy implementations and the involvement of every single layer of the government branch. The fundamental objective is to create an unsympathetic environment for plague and an unfavorable environment for the virus to live and spread.

Furthermore, fighting a pandemic requires specific short and long-term efforts by various departments of the government. State-society cooperation is needed in a way to win this never-ending battle. Strategically, response to pandemic consists of bilateral and cross-discipline initiatives including state-community engagements and technology-based new-lifestyles for the prevention of expanding this deadly virus. Therefore, the COVID-19 response is an effort to help build a social resilience against COVID-19. Major cities around the world are currently struggling to deal with the COVID-19 pandemic. Some are still under full or partial lockdown, some are beginning to relax restrictions to restart their economy and social lives, while others are dealing with new waves of infections. However, the new normal is more than just practicing physical distancing and self-hygiene. It also requires us to relook at how we have been managing our countries, cities, and society, i.e. people, resources, and economy.

This book has come in place with the main agenda of generating a collection of strategies in response to COVID-19. It has outlined and detailed the necessary steps required in forming a successful program which will be demonstrated by thematic and country-based case studies. This book is aimed at providing a theoretical framework supported by case studies in various sectors. Hence, many country-based case studies on pre- and post-COVID-19 response and real-time experiences for countries in various settings are illustrated. This book serves to reinforce the framework which has been established and give a better understanding of the challenges encountered in translating theory into practice. In essence, it aims to send the message that the best ideas should be brought into perspective when crafting the right COVID-19 response. With superlative modifications, it provides an expansion of ideas for those who desire to design and implement fast and precise responses.

During peaceful times, which all countries in the world experienced prior to the outbreak of COVID-19, most countries did not put any effort into maintaining and improving the security of food and health industries. Actually, initiatives on those efforts could have been launched as early as possible, at the very beginning of the outbreak. The People's Republic of China had identified a new type of virus known as the Wuhan Virus since December 2019 and the emergence of the pandemic itself took off at the beginning of 2020. Unfortunately, the outbreak of the virus started to greatly impact the country by the end of January 2020 and forced the Chinese government to implement a total lockdown at the beginning of February 2020. As a result, people throughout the world started to learn about the deadly virus, later known as Coronavirus, and soon after, the virus spread all over the globe. The outbreak of the virus had been so massive that the World Health Organization (WHO) should have declared it as a pandemic. For the sake of practicality in dealing with the pandemic, the WHO officially named the Coronavirus as COVID-19 based on the fact that the virus refers to the Coronavirus that has been identified in 2019. In the present time, the virus, which will be referred to as COVID-19, has impacted 200 countries around the world except the ones located in the islands of the Pacific Ocean such as Tonga, Niue, Kiribati, Solomon Islands, and North Korea (Adriana, 2020).

The impact of COVID-19 is greatly perceived by every country in the world and results in the fact that defense is no longer a domain that should be given significant attention. Now, the focus of almost all governments has turned into the security of the food and health industries, as well as the reconstruction of economics (Muhyiddin, 2020). With regards to the statement, indeed there are many that should be discussed especially in terms of mitigating the impacts of COVID-19. The discussions over these aspects are highly significant since now all governments will certainly foresee a devastating economic recession that can result in a high level of poverty even in the global scale. The situation will be worse because it is possible that the rate of unemployment will increase dramatically while the gap of poverty from one community to another, and even from one country to another, will be significantly larger. Above all, the world community should live in a new-normal condition in which air travel and cross-border journals become fewer, and physical distancing and hygiene become a new set of life priorities. At the same time, work-from-home, which has been popularly abbreviated into WFH, becomes a new alternative together with online learning, which urges the schools and universities to quickly fit themselves into the new world of online teaching-learning activities. Despite the various impacts of COVID-19, the present article will focus on the impacts of COVID-19 on the aspects of global security (Muhyiddin, 2020).

With regards to the objective of the article, at least eight main impacts on global security have been identified. These eight impacts can be categorized as follows: (1) breakup groups; (2) terrorism; (3) defense industry; (4) cyber security; (5) food security; (6) health security; (7) local crimes; and (8) cross-border crimes. The eight aspects of security indeed have positive and negative impacts on all countries across the globe without any exception, even for the countries that have not been impacted by the COVID-19 outbreak. For example, the world's superpower countries have started to change their foreign policies for the very first time in order to preserve the internal security (Waxman and Wilson, 2020). The changes on the foreign policy itself can be considered very vital since COVID-19 has caused a massive number of casualties, which exceed the ones found in the history of, for instance, the Korean and Vietnam wars. Furthermore, the changes on the foreign policy made by these countries provide the best description on how COVID-19 has impacted the world; thus, these changes require all governments to re-evaluate their policies of security in place. In sum, there is one single question that should be raised in this situation: Which aspect is of utmost importance in ensuring the security of a country?

About the chapters

The threat and response of COVID-19 emerged in every aspect of modern social life, and whether we like it or not, it has given a significant impact on the whole of mankind. Numerous local and international issues including health security, food security, trans-border crime, and many more were recorded during the spread of this pandemic. Stakeholders often look for space and opportunity to manipulate the COVID-19 situation to obtain profit. Even though generally, a decline in crime rates is recorded, it is still happening and becoming more creative. Criminals will always be a step ahead in their activities (Special Branch, 2020). Wherever there is a demand, there will be supply. Each individual needs money to make a living; so do criminals.

With regards to the crime during a pandemic, the delivery of drugs using drones has been recorded in Brazil and England. Various drug consumption and wild parties take place privately by using several applications that can be downloaded on smartphones. Prostitution activities still carry on by using delivery services and many more. Even online gambling syndicates, pornography, online scams, and others continue to expand during the COVID-19 season (Special Branch, 2020). This evidently indicates that threat to security still takes place despite COVID-19 being spread in a country and among its nationals. Many countries have empowered access to the internet to fill up the boredom of staying at home. Although many use this facility for educational activities and additional knowledge, there are also those who abuse the available facilities. Numerous reports also illustrate how online scams quickly spread. Many are deceived with various websites and fake applications created. Every new product created by the government will surely be created on fake websites to confuse people, just like it happens in Malaysia, Thailand, Indonesia, Brazil, and America. Communities who spend a lot of time on the computer or use the internet are powerful targets of this group of scammers.

Cross-border crimes are also widely recorded during the COVID-19 season. Numerous crimes related to illegal immigrants, drug smuggling (contraband), firearms, human trafficking, and many more are recorded during COVID-19 (Aslam, 2020). Countries that are often targets of immigrants such as Greece, Cyprus, England, Malaysia, and Australia continue to record an increase in illegal immigrants. These criminals are not afraid of virus. They are more concerned with profits from hidden luxurious businesses which do not demand a big capital. It is a modern form of slavery that happens in many areas of the world today. This syndicate sees good space and opportunity, as a result of limited observation in the borders and entrance of a country.

Other than that, the entry of an immigrant or illegal immigrant is also believed to give a security impact when they bring in a virus with them. They actually have high potentials in bringing COVID-19 or whatever virus to countries entered. The virus will spread among them and subsequently to the general public with whom they are in physical contact. In the end, a country's safety is put in danger and exposed to socio and economic destruction.

Subsequently, the security threat during the COVID season is related to the spread of false news. Many countries have to tighten their law or create a new act to hinder the spread of false news and information, particularly concerning COVID-19 (Ministry of Defence, 2020). All sorts of false information spread in many countries has resulted in panic among the people. The government is forced to mobilize the army, police, and certain assets in order to control the instability that occurs. It is therefore necessary for a country to create a specific set of rules in order to stop the spread of false news and overcome the group better known as the 'keyboard warriors," which is a group in search of publicity from the difficulties of others (Aslam, 2019).

Criminal threat due to COVID is also related to hackers. This group sees the whole world migrating from a conventional system to the internet or an online-based system. The use of various open-source platforms has put the security data system of a certain agency or country into a dangerous position. There are government agencies that use open platforms because they lack preparation to face the COVID-19 threat. As a result, some agencies are attacked and their data platforms are hacked (Adel, 2018). This situation will be more dangerous if private information leaks and falls into the hands of the enemy or certain parties that will make it as "ransomware" (Aslam, 2019).

By integrating the right response into the pandemic, governments can engage every single department, private agency, and community to rebuild the economy and strengthen the society. Prompt responses that can be taken by governments are to stop air, water, and land traffic flow, followed by massive health tests. Secondly, compulsory quarantine or self-quarantine has to be implemented. Later countries evolve to a period called "damage control." Once the economy stops, significant consequences can be seen; the hike in the price of groceries, recession, job loss, and many more. Governments have no choice other than to respond accordingly. Stimulus packages are injected by all of the countries to regenerate the economy and help their society. Incentives are given to local SMEs to ensure that the poverty line increases at reasonable numbers. There are also several other responses including the rising numbers of digitalization in the economy and beverage sectors. The booming of "online" business and education is unstoppable and recognized as the new normal. The migration of traditional lifestyle to digital is marked by COVID-19. Hence, ten chapters have been written to give more understanding about global impact and early response throughout the entire world.

COVID-19 Pandemic: The Threat and Response focuses on the early stages of a global pandemic. In our endeavor to return to normalcy, we identify best practices including the idea of building an equitable and sustainable world. It is divided into two main sections, which are thematic and country study. The ten thematic chapters cover economy, social, politics, security, health, digital, and bioterrorism. The country studies range by continents from the United States to the Middle East and South Asia to Southeast Asia.

The book begins with Chapter 1, where Prof Rohan Gunaratna discusses how terrorist groups justify their actions by convincing their followers that Coronavirus is a signal from God and meant to exact retribution on the "other." Islamic State loyalists spout propaganda about COVID-19 being a sign that "God is against non-Muslims" while these extremists use this narrative to "legitimize calamities and justify attacks." Rohan talks about how a terrorist who manipulated the COVID-19 is a "Soldier of Allah," sent to kill disbelievers. In this chapter, Rohan also explains the COVID-19 emergence, which was in late January 2020 and started with the story that the virus is God's retribution for China's ill-treatment of Uighur. To support God's punishment, the Indonesian terrorists and their supporters called for attacks against Chinese nationals and targeted China's interests. When the virus reached Iran, the Islamic State and Al-Qaeda said God is punishing Shia Iran for fighting the Islamic caliphate and joining Bashar al-Assad, respectively. When the virus started to kill Europeans and Americans, the Islamic State said it is the retribution for the "Holocaust of Baghouz," the last territorial stronghold of the Islamic State.

Mizan Aslam, in Chapter 2, examines the impact of COVID-19 is greatly felt by every country, resulting in the importance of defense being no longer significant. The focus of the world now is more directed toward health and food safety, as well as the redevelopment of the economic sector. There are indeed many aspects regarding COVID-19 to be discussed. The world foresees a devastating economic recession that results in many countries becoming poor. The rate of unemployment will increase drastically and the poverty gap will become bigger. The world community will live in a new-normal, work-from-home to become a new alternative, online learning migration for schools and universities to become more preferable, and many more. Nonetheless, this article will focus on the effects of COVID-19 on global safety aspects. Professor Mizan also discusses eight main effects of global safety that have been identified. This includes (1) breakup groups, (2) terrorism, (3) defense industry, (4) cyber security, (5) food security, (6) health security, (7) local crimes, and (8) across border crimes. These eight aspects of safety have positive and negative impacts on all the countries in the world, without exception. World superpowers also, for the first time, have changed their external policies to the internal safety of their respective countries. In fact, the effect of COVID-19 has caused massive deaths exceeding a few vital wars in history such as the Korean and Vietnam wars. This clearly shows how COVID-19 has affected the whole world, requiring them to re-evaluate the safety policy owned by them, which is of utmost importance in ensuring the safety of a nation.

In Chapter 3, former advisor of World Bank, Dr Nihal Pitigala, examines the potential economic consequences of COVID-19 for developing countries; in particular how international trade can transmit the economic crisis across borders, drawing on the lessons learned from past crises, even if imperfect in design or scope. The trade-related transmission mechanisms unveil a mix of policy levers that may shorten the depth and duration of the unfolding economic downturn and the impact on developing economies and their citizens. COVID-19 as a global pandemic poses an unprecedented challenge to public health on a global scale, with cases now confirmed in more than 210 countries by the end of April 2020. As governments are scrambling to safeguard people's health, the contagion has fast extended to the economic sphere, creating an international economic crisis. Just as COVID-19 is unparalleled in our lifetime, in terms of its contagion rate and the toll on human lives, it is likewise unique in the expected economic contagion that is fundamentally different from and is likely to surpass previous shocks, such as the global financial crisis of 2008–09 and may even match the Great Depression. As many countries have resorted to imposing social distancing and other drastic measures to contain the pandemic, business activities have come to a virtual standstill outside of essential goods and services. Previous economic crises manifested either as demand shocks with one epicenter, such as the United States during both the global financial crisis and the Great Depression or as supply-shock, such as the 1970's OPEC oil embargo. There have been other localized mini-shocks such as the 2011 earthquake and tsunami in Japan, which triggered a supply shock that disrupted global value chains (GVCs), particularly the automotive, computer, and consumer electronics producers that rely heavily on Japanese suppliers of specialized parts and components. Despite massive stimulus packages being crafted as economic lifelines in some developed economies, global income this year is likely to shrink dramatically, with significant transmission effects to developing and emerging markets.

In Chapter 4, Thomas Wuchte and Sophie Drake mention that the greatest security challenges to humankind are not always traditional warfare or terrorism (though of course these remain significant considerations, and will only be exacerbated by COVID-19), but health crises, rising poverty, and climate change. These are not only threat multipliers, exacerbating existing inequalities and unrest, but also they bring with them a vast range of unprecedented security issues for which our multilateral organizations are either unprepared or not placing at the forefront of their agenda. Multilateral institutions must therefore be repurposed, while reprioritizing their security focus toward the imminent but harder to measure threats of the future. Multilateral organizations such as NATO and the OSCE ought to reconsider their spending priorities, which remain focused on traditional "hard" security issues such as military prepared-ness and non-proliferation, arms control, disarmament, and counter-terrorism. Threats such as these, while significant, can no longer be first among our mul-tilateral security priorities. They must now give way to the unmitigable threats (if attitudes are not changed and actions not taken) of a changing climate and extreme weather, global health emergencies, and rampant poverty. The world has needed a cohesive global response to the COVID-19 pandemic. However, multilateral institutions were not ready for this kind of non-traditional security nexus. Typically, health and climate crises have not been at the forefront of mul-tilateral security agendas and, if present, the plans put in place have not worked in practice. This pandemic is an opportunity to change the dialogue surround-ing national security priorities and to re-assess the distribution of resources accordingly. Our imminent priorities must equally be: tackling climate change, lifting developing countries out of poverty, and treating future health crises as security issues.

In Chapter 5, Dr Chandra Nilanga Samarasinghe discusses the COVID-19 pandemic as not just being a disaster; it taught many lessons to the people to think about social and economic norms of modern civilization, the pros and cons of globalization, and the importance of developing as a whole (population within the country and globally as well). Lessons of equality and equity and usefulness of sending a rocket to the moon before fulfilling the basic require-ments of the people are also discussed. Most scholars are in the opinion that the post-pandemic era will not be the continuation of the pre-pandemic era. They would like to name the situation "extraordinary" and the post-pandemic era as a "new normal world." The new normal world composes of two episodes: (1) The period until the herd immunity will develop naturally or by a vaccine and (2) the period after the herd immunity develops. When the social distancing restrictions are lifted, the world would not go back to the pre-2020 era theo-retically. The implications adapted to the system to combat the Corona pan-demic, proven advantageous and economically cost-effective, will be continued like work from home, online deals, and communication, some leisure activities, gig economic activities.

Dr Rasitha Wickramasinghe, in Chapter 6, focuses on COVID-19 as a change agent of global scale. It is an unprecedented event that forced the global econ-omy to shut down for several months with families confined to their homes. Driven by these unique circumstances, individuals, communities, businesses, and governments found new ways to go about their daily activities. The major-ity of these changes were enabled by digital technology because of the physical distancing forced on us by the COVID-19 virus. In this chapter, we explore the role played by digital technology in facilitating some of the behavioral changes, and how COVID-19 can become an accelerator for digital adoption. Dr Rasitha also explains that the whole journey of digitalization since the 1900s till now, while focusing on the last three decades; the unprecedented digital adoption has taken place in spite of pandemics (SARS and MERS outbreaks), economic crises (crash of the dot com bubble in 2000 and global financial crisis in 2008) and continued geopolitical instabilities (9/11 terror attacks, Iraq War, Brexit, US-China trade war, etc.).

Dr Animesh Roul, in Chapter 7, precisely examines the religious congregation as a catalyst of spreading COVID-19 in the Indian subcontinent. This unprecedented pandemic has certainly exposed myriad vulnerabilities of the modern world, severely questioning the so-called human progress in the sphere of scientific innovations and advances in the global health care system. It also exposed the socio-religious divide and defiance within communities and lack of collective responsibilities in the face of this gargantuan challenge before the humanity at present. Amid this unprecedented global calamity, obstinate and opportunistic ultra-conservative religious groups willfully resisted and defied prescribed norms made to restrict the horizontal spread of the deadly pathogen. Similar to the Islamist jihadi forces who have blatantly celebrated the deaths and destruction due to the spread of the disease, terming the virus as "divine solider" or "divine retribution," several mainstreams but orthodox religious institutions observed the virus as a God sent force and it is playing havoc due to widespread disobedience to God and increasing human sins on this earth. These conservative religious groups and subgroups (Muslim, Jewish, and Christian) have invoked eschatological belief such as "Day of Judgement" to justify it as "God given phenomena" and only "He" can help the humanity from this disaster, and prayer is the last resort for survival. These groups and their spiritual leaders showed irresponsible behavior and sometimes willful negligence to exacerbate the virus spread, complicating the fight against the pandemic with their superstitions and blind belief in their respective supreme entities. Dr Roul, in this chapter highlights the controversial and rather critical role of religious and faith-based congregations in the South Asian region, especially in India, Pakistan, Sri Lanka, and Bangladesh, in transmitting or spreading the virus, either intentionally or inadvertently defying pandemic-specific regulations. Fortunately, Bangladesh escaped unscathed from the COVID-19 spike due to large gatherings but the rest of the three countries of South Asia have experienced more or less a COVID-19 spike due to the unrestricted and sometimes deliberate religious gatherings or congregations that exacerbated the COVID-19 cases substantially and even proved fatal. The paper also examines how the activities of these communities' religious groups and institutions that defy government directives of lockdown and social distancing have accelerated virus transmissions and compromised the safety and security of others.

In Chapter 8, Dr Rusdi Omar and Dr Knocks Tapiwa Zengeni converse on the implications of the COVID-19 on the ASEAN security community. Dr Rusdi and Dr Knocks propose that the ASEAN and its member states should work together to reinforce national healthcare systems and contain the spread of future communicable viruses. At the same time, the ASEAN and its member states should develop strategies of resilience and governance that may mitigate the socioeconomic impact of global health pandemics and epidemics. The ASEAN's response to global health pandemics should thus focus on key priorities such as limiting the spread of the diseases, ensuring the provision of medical equipment, promoting research for treatments and vaccines as well as providing a compassionate environment supporting jobs, businesses, and the economies of member states. The essence of our argument is that regional cooperation in non-traditional security in ASEAN should be deepened. But now, there is a much more basic question about whether regional blocs can protect the citizens of their member states from pandemics. Through consensus, contingency planning, and coordination, the ASEAN regional bloc can provide a unity of effort to advance cooperative security. This more effective, efficient, and supporting environment is a foundational step necessary to create a more resilient region better able to address the challenges of global pandemics of the present and into our future. This chapter will thus interrogate ASEAN's cooperative security in the context of regional, sub-regional, and national policy strategies to address a transnational threat of communicable diseases. To be more specific, both authors' objective is to understand how ASEAN-centered regionalism may evolve in the post-COVID-19 era, as it addresses emerging threats of the 21st century. In other words, whether the COVID-19 global health crisis provided the stimulus for institutional development in ASEAN community.

Shane Britten, in Chapter 9, canvasses terrorism and biological weapons. The terrorists' narrative of using COVID-19 as bioterrorism can be denied. We cannot discount the possibility of a group like the Islamic State attempting to use COVID-19 as a weapon. It fits the group's narrative of inflicting God's wrath on unbelievers, and creates a culture of fear, uncertainty, and economic damage; all positive outcomes for the group. What it does not fit, however, is the individual motivation and personal narrative for many extremists. If the virus is a punishment, why does it not discriminate with whom it infects? It changes the extremist from a soldier seeking to carry out an attack, to the more extreme end of terrorism and potentially carrying out a suicide attack. But where the structure of radicalization for a suicide bomber is quite well established in the Islamic State, it is a different psychological process to convince an individual to conduct an attack using a bioweapon where they are the attack vectors. Shane Britten also discusses lessons learned from COVID-19, this pandemic taught us that our governments need to be better at sharing and cross-referencing data between agencies, including those not traditionally inside the national or homeland security apparatus. It is only through this data sharing and correlation that agencies will be able to identify individual extremists becoming associated with those being tested or confirmed positive, and conduct urgent investigations on whether this is a deliberate act with the intent of consciously spreading the virus. Our agencies must have access to streamlined systems, processes, and tracking of cases to identify their origin and method of contracting the disease. This is difficult at a time when the virus has crippled economies around the world, but without investing in the infrastructure needed to facilitate information exchange and correlation, the impact of the virus is likely to be more severe for a longer period of time.

In the final chapter, Richard Chasdi presents an update on enhanced terrorism and the prospect of its use in the United States. Professor Chasdi expands the concept of "enhanced terrorism," a condition whereby terrorism is used with enhanced effects amid calamitous chemical, biological, radiological, or nuclear (CBRN) conditions. The framework for discussion by Chasdi involves a description of enhanced terrorism's "proactive" and "ad-hoc" dimensions; heuristically driven extensions of the conceptualization's implications and applications; description about terrorist groups splintering or in cohesion conditions and trajectories within calamitous conditions. The concept of "enhanced terrorism" is articulated with two subtypes: (1) "proactive" enhanced terrorism and (2) "ad-hoc" enhanced terrorism. In the case of "proactive" enhanced terrorism, terrorist group leaders use traditional terrorism and cyberterrorism to take advantage of calamitous conditions to enhance terrorist assault effects. In the post-corona virus era, what is implicitly understood in the carefully reasoned terrorism planning that is the hallmark of "proactive" enhanced terrorism, is the potential for enhanced terrorism to have compound ripple effects across environmental system dimensions with direct and indirect connections. In the United States, many of the motivations that drive closer affiliation to political movements that promote social equality and economic justice are linked to anger, frustration, and similar sentiments about political, economic, cultural, and social disparities between communities in society. A calamitous condition such as Coronavirus works to sharpen those differences, and those motivational demands that lead political movement affiliations can, if left unattended, increase the potential for terrorism. This resonates with Gurr's notion of "relative deprivation theory," where more plentiful economic and political opportunities associated with one particular ethnic, racial, or religious group stand in such stark relief to the limited opportunities of other groups, that the likelihood of armed conflict in a country increases. Hence, the potential for enhanced terrorism is not necessarily limited to "right-wing" political groups, but includes "left-wing" political groups fighting to ensure access and availability. Under such calamitous conditions, non-violent political movements are vulnerable to the prospect of group fragmentation, where political movements can spawn terrorist group splinters or spinoff groups within the context of inadequate government response to political demands and aspirations.

Conclusion

The world is in an enormous crisis. Since the Second World War ended, most countries in the world had been in their comfort zones and were not prepared to face threats like this. The spread of COVID-19, which was then announced as a pandemic by WHO, startled the world and is now in search of the best remedy to handle it. Every party that argues has to return to the discussion table and agree to take action to stop the current conflict.

Every nation has to collaborate and those in conflict must build good cooperation amongst each other so that the conflict can be put to a stop. Regions under conflict such as the Middle East and South Asia, as well as Latin America, have connections with other countries. The conflict requires cooperation between governments in order to end it. The success of handling a crisis will not happen with the effort of only one party; it requires the involvement of various sincere and committed parties. It is not necessary to have hidden agendas when handling conflicts at this time because a bigger effect concerning COVID-19 needs to be thought out.

Cooperation from various Non-Governmental Agencies (NGO) and also Civil Society Organizations (CSO) is essential and can be moved now. Initiatives of country-community and government-private taken such as in Yemen and Asia too seem to be a noble effort. Today, the success of handling COVID-19 is not only put on one particular country or government. It however appears as a collective step by involving various agencies including NGO and CSO, which have the same objectives, which are to end the disputes and consequently overcome the COVID-19 threat. Every party, including influential individuals from religious groups, women, and the local leaders can also be moved in order to end all forms of conflict in the world today.

COVID-19 has made it extremely challenging to convene conflict parties in direct negotiations. It will not deter the whole world from pursuing best conflict solutions. We must be creative and shall use the latest technology such as IoT and Big Data to the maximum extent possible to maintain open channels of communications and de-escalate the conflict. These initiatives need to be supported by pro-active diplomatic engagement and action. It is a big task to bring the voices of other actors including NGO, CSO, religious leaders, women, youth, and every single unit of people, in our efforts to secure sustainable agreements to uphold international peace and security.

References

Aslam, M.M. (2019). Artificial Intelligence (AI) Belum Cukup Bagus. Special Column in Harian Metro, 13th June 2019. Kuala Lumpur: Media Prima.

Aslam, M.M. (2020). Pemahaman Agama Ketika Wabak. Terbitan Malaysiakini pada 11 April 2020. Retrieved on the 11th April 2020 from: https://www.malaysiakini.com/columns/520063

Gunaratna, R. (2020). TAG COVID-19 Briefing. Washington: The Asia Group.

Interview with Perlis Special Branch Director, Royal Malaysia Police. Dated: 06th of May 2020.

Kalbana, P., and Chan, D. (2020, 2 Mei). A Longer Wait Could Have Resulted in More Losses in Revenue. Retrieved on the 03rd of May 2020 from: New Straits Times: https://www.nst.com.my/news/nation/2020/05/589227/longer-wait-could-have-resulted-more-losses-revenue pada 2 Mei 2020

Ministry of Defence. (2020). Kekang PATI, Keselamatan Negara Terus Diperketat, Kawal Pendatang. Dilayari pada 27 April 2020 dari laman sesawang: http://www.mod.gov.my/ms/mediamenu/berita/701-kekang-pati-kawalan-sempadan-negara-terus-diperketat-diperhebat

Muhyiddin, Mohd Yassin (2020, 1 Mei). Teks Perutusan Khas YAB Tan Sri Dato' Haji Muhyiddin bin Haji Mohd Yassin, Perdana Menteri Malaysia sempena Hari Pekerja. Putrajaya: Pejabat Perdana Menteri.

Rodriguez, Adriana. (2020). These Countries Have No Reports on Coronavirus Cases. But Can They be Trusted?. Retrieved on the 07th of May 2020 from: https://www.usatoday.com/story/news/world/2020/05/06/covid-19-which-countries-have-no-coronavirus-cases/3076741001/

Waxman, O., and Wilson, C. (2020). How The Coronavirus Death Toll Compares to Other Deadly Events From American History. Retrieved on the 30th of April 2020 from: https://time.com/5815367/coronavirus-deaths-comparison/

1 Terrorism amid a pandemic

Rohan Gunaratna

Introduction

The coronavirus, known officially as SARS-CoV-2 (COVID-19), is an apex and an evolving threat. As the virus spreads and mutates, the threat groups are exploring and exploiting the pandemic to advance their agenda. Although lockdowns inhibit attacks in government-controlled areas, terrorist attacks continue unabated in the conflict areas. While government entities and military forces abide by lockdown measures, postponing training and scaling down operations, insurgent and terrorist groups operate relatively freely in mounting attacks. Both in the battlefields and off-the-battlefields, threat groups invest in digital acceleration, maintaining strength and ideological influence during COVID-19.

From disseminating propaganda to raising funds, these threat groups foment racial and religious tension and violence. By engaging in such support activity, terrorist and extremist groups fuel the recruiting momentum. They link up online with like-minded groups and build communities of supporters and sympathizers. The religious fanatics argue that COVID-19 is a "soldier of God," "a divine retribution," and waging "Corona jihad" to infect opponents. While Muslim fanatics advocate infecting Muslim officials and non-Muslims, Far Right (Extreme Right Wing: XRW) advocated direct action of deliberately spreading the virus to "non-whites" – minorities and immigrants. The ethnopolitical groups lobby to build support and influence both at home and abroad.

With the COVID-19 developing into a global pandemic, terrorist ideologies and extremist thinking influence the human terrain. The ideologies of violent groups also fuse with the thinking of political parties bolstering each other. The Far-Right groups influence a segment of the general population against migrants, immigration, and people of color and minorities. The Far-Right groups and Republicans in the United States feed off each other. The Muslim threat entities politicize, radicalize and mobilize segments of communities to use the virus to their advantage to target their adversaries. The Muslim threat groups and Islamists parties feed off each other, affirming the terrorism–political nexus.

Easily accessible and relatively low-risk bioweapon, rapidly transmitted and inconspicuously spread, will threat certain groups to weaponize COVID-19

DOI: 10.4324/9781003197416-1

for their own benefits. Considering that younger and less susceptible assailants can be used to infect older and vulnerable populations, will they deliberately spread COVID-19 in target communities and countries? Considering the recent developments, the concern of the security and intelligence community is real. The governments and community partners need to monitor the evolving ideologies and operational capabilities of a spectrum of threat groups and personalities.

The context

A small number of threat groups with access to resources have expressed an interest to develop and use biological and other weapons of mass destruction (WMD).[1] Will the pandemic instigate or inspire Islamic State and Al Qaeda, the two most powerful insurgent and terrorist groups in the world, to invest in WMD stealth programs?

Since the 1990s, a few threat groups invested in chemical, biological, radiological and nuclear (CBRN) programs. They recruited or coerced scientists to build programs to weaponize anthrax, botulinum, Ebola, and other forms of viruses and bacteria. Governments disrupted some of these secret programs by targeting their facilities and killing or capturing rogue scientists. The others did not materialize due to the lack of terrorist technical and manufacturing capacities. Among the challenges of the terrorist projects face is gaining access to pathogens and vaccines to protect their own members.

Since the beginning of the contemporary wave of terrorism in 1979, there has not been so much chatter on a virus. Worldwide terrorist groups have expressed interest in COVID-19. Bad actors have already engaged in its malicious spread, particularly within law enforcement and medical research facilities. In the UK, infected assailants used spit as a weapon on police officers. A spokeswoman for the Police Federation said:

> We have seen some vile and disgusting acts by a minority, weaponising Covid-19 by spitting and coughing at officers. It is therefore absolutely right and proper that the home secretary is clear that those who do so should feel the full weight of the law. Those responsible for weaponising the virus are the lowest of the low.[2]

Belly Mujinga, a 47-year-old British railway ticket office worker, died after a man deliberately coughed on her. Transport Salaried Staffs' Association said:

> She is one of far too many frontline workers who have lost their lives to coronavirus.[3]

In Belgium, where several cases of spitting are reported, offenders could be fined up to €2,400 and could face prison terms up to two years. If claiming to be infected to scare others, the offenders will be subjected to the same penalties.[4]

A Pennsylvania woman Margaret Cirko, 35-year-old, coughed and spit on US$35,000 worth of produce and merchandise at a grocery store. Arrested and charged with two felony counts of terrorist threats, one felony count of threats to use a "biological agent" and one felony count of criminal mischief, she reportedly said:

> I have the virus. Now everyone is going to get sick.[5]

Although the virus is hard to weaponize except one to one infection, an assailant could infect VIPs, security, or frontline officials.

To 143,195 followers on Facebook on March 1, 2020, New York-based Muslim Brotherhood activist Bahgat Saber called for Egyptians to intentionally infect government officials and state employees on his Facebook page.

> If you are a soldier, you can go into the defense ministry, and shake hands with all the generals of the military and the police. The same is true with the justice system.

On a Facebook live session, Saber incited,

> If you have contracted coronavirus, you should exact revenge! Avenge yourself, avenge the honor of your women, avenge the people who are in prison, and avenge the oppressed people. Go there. Why die alone? When you die, why die alone?[6]

Background

The terrorist interest in COVID-19 can be traced back to the outbreak in Wuhan in China in January 2020. The very first COVID-19 post by a terrorist group was by the supporters of the Islamic State monitoring the developments in Xinjiang, China. With hundreds of Uighur fighters in Syria and Afghanistan, Islamic State and their supporters regularly expressed their views with regard to the developments in Xinjiang. On January 27, 2020, a poster designed and distributed by Quraysh Media depicted a person in a gas mask at the forefront and a city in the background. The English text reading: "China Coronavirus," "A promise is a debt that we must not forget," and "Quraysh Media 2020" was superimposed on the artwork. Although the pro-Islamic State media did not identify the "promise," supporters exposed to Islamic State propaganda saw it as revenge for China's persecution of Uyghur Muslims. In the northwest Xinjiang province, the Chinese response to terrorism was to integrate the indigenous Uighurs with Han settlers, Uighur re-education (mainstream through rehabilitation), and enforce strict measures to restore local and traditional Islam by regulating the Islamic space. The theme, Wuhan coronavirus and its outbreak in China as a punishment for the country, was repeated until the virus evolved from an endemic to an epidemic. After having afflicted the Chinese, with the virus spreading from China to other countries, the Islamic State narrative changed. When the virus afflicted Iran, the Islamic State supporters said Iranian Shia are being punished for its "idolatry." When the virus spread to Europe and the United States, the Islamic State supporters said, Europeans and Americans were punished for being "polytheist nations."

Echoing Islamic State belief of the virus being a blessing from Allah, created as a form of punishment, the theme reverberated among a segment of Muslims even after the virus was declared a global pandemic. The Islamist thinking of depicting natural disasters as God's will continues. In the eyes of the Muslim threat groups, the virus did not infect believers. The March 19, 2020, *Al Naba* [dispatch] editorial titled "The Crusaders' Worst Nightmare," reports "Fear of this contagion has affected them more than the contagion itself."[7]

Al Qaeda, Islamic State and its affiliates exploited the COVID-19 situation to expand their geographic footprint. Within the followers, rank and file of Al Qaeda and Islamic State, they are increasingly propagating the message that COVID-19 is infecting the disbelievers and shielding the Muslim believers. With COVID-19 infecting large segments of the Chinese, Iranian, and western public, Al Qaeda and Islamic State followers said that COVID-19 is celestial punishment. Calling it divine revenge, Islamic State supporters said

> it is the prayer of the people of Baghouz whom you burnt alive. It has killed you. So reap the results of your actions.[8]

Portraying the coronavirus as divine retribution, Al-Azm Media Foundation published the 15 minute, 38 second video, entitled, "And None Can Know the Hosts of Your Lord but He," on May 18, 2020. In its production, Al-Azm features clips from past Islamic State (IS) videos, showing fighters in Baghouz, Syria, bombs falling on IS-held territories, and an English-speaking fighter celebrating the disasters from Hurricanes Irma and Harvey in the United States, and footage from news media concerning people who died from COVID-19, to argue that the virus was sent by God to punish Western states and their allies and other foes for what befell Muslims. It then displays infographics on infections and deaths in the United States, Spain, Russia, Britain, Italy, France, Germany, Iran, China, Belgium, and Israel. Islamic State, Al-Qaeda and supporting groups compared the impact of COVID-19 on its enemies. Stating that America isn't all-powerful and invincible, the Islamic State pointed that in one week more Americans died of COVID-19 infection than the nearly 3,000 killed on 9/11.

> It is falsehood to worship America and to fear it instead of Allah the Almighty.[9]

Al-Qaeda propaganda arm As-Sahab said:

> Allah, the Creator, has revealed the brittleness and vulnerability of your material strength. It is now clear for all to see that it was but a deception

that could not stand the test of the smallest soldier of God on the face of the earth.[10]

The very idea that the virus is "soldier of Allah" grew worldwide among threat groups and supporters. Describing the Virus as "Army of Allah" and "the smallest army of Allah," "Balik I.," a radical convert in the Philippines, posted a Facebook message on May 19, 2020, and again on May 21, 2020, posted another message claiming that Muslims in Mindanao are not doing anything to stop the abuses of the "kuffar" (infidels) and mocked them for not taking action.[11]

Most terrorist groups and their followers defied quarantine restrictions from mosque closures and lockdown measures. They incited attacks during the COVID-19 pandemic. To their advantage, the safety precautions required to prevent infection were neglected by the threat groups. Balik I.'s account continued to assert that, unlike shopping malls that are already open, Mosques are being kept closed because no one is fighting for it. Balik I. then urged its followers to engage in violence by stating, in part:

> Being patient in the abuses of the kuffar? Brother and sisters, that is not the right kind of patience for you. Instead, be patient with the orders of Allah, that is, fight to protect Islam.[12]

In the Philippines, Islamic State supporters advocated violence to reopen mosques closed by COVID-19 restrictions.

During Ramadan (April 23–May 23, 2020), threat groups believed that there rewards for mounting attacks would be multiplied. In response to the call, both operatives and supporters threatened attacks in retaliation for closing the mosques. Two Islamic State supporters in Tunisia attempted to infect police officers by coughing and deliberately contaminating a busy precinct.

The Ministry of the Interior said, in a statement, that

> the terrorist element, who was recently released after his involvement in a case of terrorist nature, took advantage of his moral authority over the rest of the Takfiri elements in the region, especially those who have symptoms of the emerging coronavirus and who are under administrative control in order to incite them to intentionally sneeze and cough and spread spit everywhere, while they are inside the security centre.[13]

The Tabligh Jamaat, a movement of conservative Muslims, held congregations throughout Asia despite government and other warnings.[14]

Although the media focus has been on Muslims, Christian and Jewish congregations also created COVID-19 clusters.[15] In addition to conservative Muslims, if terrorists and extremists continue to deliberately spread the virus, Islamophobic sentiments will grow. Already from India to the United Kingdom and the United States, the Far-Right thinking and ideologies advocate hatred against Muslims as "super spreaders."

In the eyes of the threat groups and their supporters, the enemies of Allah suffered. They are beginning to believe the virus mostly attacked infidels (unbelievers) and apostates (renounced belief). In their eyes, the Chinese suffered due to its mistreatment of Uighurs, Iran due to the role of its Shia, and the West (Europe and the United States) due to their interventions, especially in Iraq and Syria. Those indoctrinated said COVID-19 is revenge for Muslim lives lost in Baghouz, the last territorial stronghold of the Islamic State in Syria that was bombed by the coalition airstrikes. The question in their mind is whether there is still a need to weaponize COVID-19 to enhance God's wrath on its enemies.

Far-Right groups

The virus drew the attention of a spectrum of threat groups. Contrary to public perception, Far-Right groups exploited the virus more than politico-religious groups. The Far-Right discourse paints national governments and international institutions as either responsible for or complicit in the spread of COVID-19. Far-Right commentators from France, Italy, and Spain converge on the notion that official responses to the pandemic have been driven by a supposedly sinister ulterior motive.[16] Directed at the private sector, the Far-Right released a clip Plandemic engendering public mistrust of health institutions. In defiance of lockdown measures from disobeying quarantine regulations and organized protests, the Far-Right measures criticize government measures to impose "authoritarian" control over populations. In addition to vandalizing NY healthcare workers' vehicles, the Far Right incited those infected to cough on healthcare workers and for nails to be placed in the hospital parking lots. Capitalizing on fears, disillusionment, and social tensions, Far-Right groups shared disinformation reaching out to their supporters and potential supporters in the surface, deep, and dark web.

Lockdown protests by harnessing antiestablishment and social discontent, Far-Right groups and supporters targeted Muslims, Jews, and Asians, especially ethnic Chinese. Singaporean law student Jonathan Mok suffered from a coronavirus-related racist attack in London on February 24, 2020. After calling Mok "coronavirus" and "I don't want your coronavirus in my country," he was punched in the face again (Clement Yong, 2020)[17] In addition to targeting Muslim and Jewish places of religious worship, their day-care centers were targeted with chemical and biological weapons by neo-Nazi members. They said the virus created a way for Jews to sell vaccines. Neo-Nazi members called on others to "spread the flu to every Jew." Neo-Nazi forum urged anyone diagnosed with the virus to cough into their hands and touch "things that will have high contact traffic [such as] door handles, handrails, restrooms, sink taps, etc." Others suggest those infected with the virus withdraw hundreds of dollars in small bills, contaminate them, and then "hit up major stores in lots of different cities." To expand their base, most Far-Right groups promoted white nationalism.

Motivated by "racial, religious and anti-government animus," Timothy Wilson, a 36-year-old white supremacist, planned to trigger an explosives-laden vehicle and detonate in the parking lot of Belton Regional Medical Center in

Cass County, Missouri, United States. Hitherto Wilson planned to hit an elementary school with African-American students, power grid, bridges, nuclear plant, Islamic centers in Missouri, synagogue in Arkansas, Walmart headquarters and the University of Kansas Hospital in Kansas City, Kansas. Injured in a shootout with the police, Wilson died on March 24, 2020. Two days earlier, Wilson visited the hospital property and conducted a dry run. Starting January 30, Wilson bought explosive precursors – two 5-pound bags of urea and 60 pounds of ammonium nitrate and another type of fertilizer. Before his separation, Wilson served the Navy and received the "E" Ribbon, Good Conduct Medal, National Defense Service Medal, Iraq Campaign Medal, Global War on Terrorism Service Medal, and Coast Guard Special Operations Service Medal.

After the Christchurch attack in 2019, the Far-Right violence in the West surpassed attacks by Muslim threat groups. This trend is likely to continue considering widespread desperation mobilizing large segments of the population. With the social dislocation and radicalization, the Far-Right has exploited the COVID-19 to grow its support base significantly from North America to Europe and Australia. To garner media attention, the Far-Right publicly identified COVID-19 as a "Chinese Virus" and welcomed the pandemic.

On February 19, 2020, an online content aggregator published in a Far-Right telegram channel "the black swan event" as an opportunity "to destabilize the kike economy (implying a Jewish controlled economy) and create the necessary conditions under which revolution is possible."[18] "The glorious Happening is upon us," read the post, referring to a race war and stoke racism toward "Asians."[19] The Far-Right channel published a list of "accelerationism goals" to be achieved by driving racial and political narratives about the outbreak. "We need to #1 racialize it and #2 politicize it. In the coming weeks I anticipate hundreds of chinks racial slur for a person of Chinese descent) and urbanites to be confirmed infected in the USA."[20] The Far-Right identifies its Accelerationism Goals as:

1 Praise the arrival of the WuFlu Pandemic loudly so that the Jew media takes notice;
2 Stigmatize Asians to exacerbate racial tensions and create fear;
3 Celebrate the climbing death counts and laugh at the suffering of the shit-libs in the cities;
4 Make comparisons to the End Times to further spread panic;
5 Encourage making necessary preparations so that the store shelves clean out and the markets crash.[21]

The sanitized strategy acceptable to the public is to weaken government by creating lockdown protests but the most extreme Far Right discussed how to turn the virus into a bio-weapon.

> "What to do if you get COVID-19", a Far Right post urged its followers, "Visit your local Mosque!, visit your local synagogue!; spend time in diverse neighbourhoods! spend the day on public transports!"[22]

In continental Europe, the uncertainty surrounding the coronavirus has led to a boom in conspiracy theories on social media. The public spending time online, especially joining conspiracy theory groups on Telegram, fueled the beliefs of such theories, said Amadeu-Antonio Anti-Racism Foundation's Miro Dittrich.[23] Dittrich said conspiracy theory topics included vaccines, contactless payment, and 5G masts.

> 5G has remained a core Coronavirus conspiracy topic for actors on the far-right and far-left alike, who posit that the cell towers are part of a plan by the faceless 'elite' to spread COVID-19.[24]

Strategic use of disease

To the current and future threat entities, the COVID-19 pandemic is the strategic use of disease as a weapon on a global scale.

The pandemic exposed the weaknesses and the strengths of the international, regional and domestic frameworks to deal with a biological threat. The pandemic tested the preparedness of the government and partners to manage a very real threat. Although it would depend on the agent, in the event of a deliberate biological attack, the impact would not be too dissimilar.

The pandemic has made threat groups aware of the threat posed by conventional and unconventional weapons. Their understanding and awareness of biological agents grew. A few threat groups such as Al Qaeda, Aum Shinrikyo, and others have experimented with biological agents. A larger number of groups such as the Islamic State and their local affiliates have expressed an interest in exploring the weapons of mass distraction spectrum.

A once-in-a-century moment

Will the COVID-19 pandemic be a once-in-a-century moment? The pandemic is unlikely to go away in the immediate or the short term (1–2 years). It is likely to persist in the mid-term (5 years). Unless the world invests in capabilities to better manage epidemics and pandemics, it is likely to witness similar threats in the foreseeable future (10 years).

It is very likely that the pandemic will continue to catalyze and stimulate some threat actors to develop biological weapons in the foreseeable future. However, most would realize the limitations of exploiting biological agents as well. As of today, most threat groups are comfortable using the proven weapons – the gun and the bomb. Nonetheless, the pandemic made the threat entities – groups, networks, cells and personalities – experience the impact of a biological threat. Had the governments acted decisively, the thinking of the threat entities would be different. It is vital for government and partners to respond effectively supported by an effective communications strategy.

A few threat entities, mostly Al Qaeda and Islamic State and their associates, were able to harness the COVID-19 narrative effectively. Although they exploited its narrative during the first half a year, it has tapered down with the virus affecting both Muslim and non-Muslim communities alike. Like the rest of the world, they continue to live through the pandemic, experiencing lockdowns, partial lockdowns and pandemic restrictions.

Likely trajectory

As the threat groups are becoming creative and innovative, governments should plan for two scenarios – the most likely and worst-case scenarios. In forecasting the worst-case scenario, the past and the present is the best guide. Although incidents of terrorists using biological agents are rare, terrorist access to rogue scientists is becoming common. If this persists, the future may be different. Until now, the most successful unconventional weapons program by a non-state actor was by Aum. The Tokyo Subway Sarin attack by Aum Shinrikyo in 1995, the most significant terrorist attack in Japan's modern history, played a key role in influencing other terrorist groups to seek technology and expertise to conduct CBRN attacks.

Aum Shinrikyo is one of the most violent groups that emerged before the rise of Al-Qaeda and the so-called Islamic State (IS). The group had long-term goals that included building conventional military strength and recruiting youth from universities and industries working on technical subjects. Aum Shinrikyo managed to evade scrutiny by using the cover of religion in support of its activities.

Both state and non-state actors have learned from Aum Shinrikyo's extensive biological and chemical programs. Aum Shinrikyo's attacks have also provided governments with a template for responding to the CBRN threat posed by groups such as IS and Al-Qaeda.

In order to support its militarization program in Japan, Aum Shinrikyo built state-of-the-art national and international procurement networks. The group built a stronghold close to Mount Fuji and other smaller factories to produce special weapons and create a chemical stockpile. The group built its biological and chemical warfare program by recruiting 300 qualified and trained Japanese scientists and engineers. The program started with Seiichi Endo, a virologist trained at Kyoto University, harvesting botulinum bacterium from the Ishikarigawa Basin in Hokkaido Prefecture in 1989.12 Aum Shinrikyo also attempted to acquire agents from overseas to build its biological warfare program. In October 1992, Aum Shinrikyo dispatched a medical mission led by Asahara to Zaire to provide aid during an Ebola outbreak, but its motive was to obtain the Ebola virus. The group procured vaccines and pathogens from Japanese universities and through followers who purchased them overseas.

The Aum Shinrikyo branch in New York attempted to obtain high technology equipment, computer software, hardware and military items. In order to handle chemical and biological agents in their 'clean rooms' in Tokyo, the group purchased air filtration media from a company in New Hampshire in 1994. In January 1995, the group's members also purchased molecular modeling software in Oregon. Some of the products purchased had enabled a chemist to synthesize molecular experimentation on a computer screen instead of in a laboratory. The downloads from other databanks were used for analysis and data modeling. Aum Shinrikyo members negotiated the purchase of a sophisticated computer hardware system to use the software for US$ 47,000 in February and March 1995. Even though Aum Shinrikyo killed 27 people in its attacks, the group was feared because its chemical attacks injured and indirectly affected over 6,000 civilians. The biological warfare program of Aum Shinrikyo was a failure, but its scientists secretly manufactured and successfully delivered nerve agents. VX was used to kill dissidents and Sarin was employed to kill judges and the public. From 1990 to 1995, the group initiated 17 attacks, which included ten chemical and seven biological attacks to target civilians and officials.

Investigations have confirmed that four biological attacks used anthrax and three used botulinum, while four chemical attacks used Sarin; four other attacks used VX, one attack used phosgene and another used hydrogen cyanide.

Just like the Aum program offers many instructive lessons on recruiting rogue scientists, Al Qaeda's anthrax program one and two inform likely future developments. Governments worldwide should pay attention to the scientists and others with access to pathogens and vaccines. They should watch both the battlefield and off-the-battlefield actors that express interest to move in the CBRN spectrum and take appropriate measures.

Conclusion

The COVID-19 pandemic changed the biothreat and risk landscape. The pandemic prompted governments and their partners to discuss the threat and risk of biological agents publicly. The pandemic built capabilities within governments and partners to better understand and respond to bio threats. Furthermore, the response to the pandemic made available to the public ready access to personal protection equipment, vaccines, testing kits and the knowledge of how governments trace the infected. Aware of government and partner deficiencies, threat entities can effectively misuse and abuse both technology and expertise to build their own special weapons programs. An extraordinary effort is needed to secure threat entities from gaining access to virulent strains of biological agents and to develop capabilities to manage likely future threats.

To prevent future mass casualty and mass fatality attacks, governments will have to work together with a range of actors – the industry, academia, private medical and health sector and community. More importantly, governments will have to work with the media and build their own strategic communications and information/influence operations capabilities.

The post-COVID-19 world will witness greater challenges for the national and international security community. National and international security leaders will have to reprioritize threats. They will need to demonstrate visionary, collective and decisive leadership when dealing with similar future threats. How governments successfully managed or failed to manage the COVID-19 pandemic will provide them the best guidance.

Notes

1. The New Arab, "Malaysia releases scientist who tried to build biological weapons for Bin Laden," November 21, 2019. https://english.alaraby.co.uk/english/news/2019/11/21/malaysia-releases-bin-ladens-anthrax-scientist
   Malaysiakini, "Yazid a member of JI Malaysia, witness tells court," October 7, 2015. https://m.malaysiakini.com/news/314941
   NBC NEWS, "Al-Qaida takes center stage in Padilla trial," June 25, 2007. http://www.nbcnews.com/id/19420820/ns/us_news-security/t/al-qaida-takes-center-stage-padilla-trial/#.XwKbiygzaiM
   Abby Goodnough, "Prosecutors turn to Padilla for closing arguments," *The New York Times*, August 14, 2007. https://www.nytimes.com/2007/08/14/us/14padilla.html
2. Matthew Weaver and Vikram Dodd, "Coronavirus outbreak, police examine CCTV footage of suspect who spat at UK rail worker who later died," *The Guardian*, May 13, 2020. https://www.google.com/amp/s/amp.theguardian.com/world/2020/may/13/police-examine-cctv-footage-of-suspect-who-spat-at-uk-rail-worker-who-later-died
3. DW, "Coronavirus: UK rail worker dies after 'carrier' spat on her," May 12, 2020. https://amp.dw.com/en/coronavirus-uk-rail-worker-dies-after-carrier-spat-on-her/a-53417624
4. The Brussels Times, "Coronavirus: Belgium makes spitting punishable by fines and jail time," March 31, 2020. https://www.brusselstimes.com/brussels/103711/coronavirus-belgium-makes-spitting-punishable-by-fines-and-jail-time/
5. James Halpin and Bob Kalinowski, "Hanover township woman charged in Gerrity's Supermarket coughing episode," *The Times-Tribune*, March 26, 2020. https://m.thetimes-tribune.com/coronavirus/hanover-township-woman-charged-in-gerritys-supermarket-coughing-episode-1.2611519
6. Ismaeel Naar, "Coronavirus: Muslim brotherhood activist calls on Egyptians to infect officials," *Al Arabiya English*, March 18, 2020. https://english.alarabiya.net/en/media/digital/2020/03/18/Coronavirus-Muslim-Brotherhood-activist-calls-on-Egyptians-to-infect-officials.html
7. International Crisis Group, "Contending with ISIS in the time of coronavirus," March 31, 2020. https://www.crisisgroup.org/global/contending-isis-time-coronavirus
8. Terrorism Research and Analysis Consortium (TRAC), "Corona: It is the prayer of the people of al-Baghouz, whom you burned alive, it has killed you so reap the results of your actions," March 23, 2020. https://www.trackingterrorism.org/chatter/cgi-green-b1rds-unofficial-islamic-state-corona-it-prayer-people-al-baghouz-whom-you-burned-
9. James Gordon Meek, "Terrorist groups spin COVID-19 as God's 'smallest soldier' attacking West," *ANC News*, April 2, 2020. https://www.google.com/amp/s/abcnews.go.com/amp/International/terrorist-groups-spin-covid-19-gods-smallest-soldier/story%3fid=69930563
10. Ibid.
11. SITE Intelligence Group, "Call for violence to reopen Philippine Mosque closed by COVID-19 restrictions," May 22, 2020. https://ent.siteintelgroup.com/Jihadist-Threat-Southeast-Asia/call-for-violence-to-reopen-philippine-mosques-closed-by-covid-19-restrictions.html
12. Ibid.
13. Middle East Monitor, "Tunisia announces failure of a 'terrorist plot' to spread coronavirus," April 17, 2020. https://www.google.com/amp/s/www.middleeastmonitor.com/20200417-tunisia-announces-failure-of-a-terrorist-plot-to-spread-coronavirus/amp/

14. Joanna Slater, Niha Masih and Shams Irfan, "India confronts its first coronavirus 'super-spreader' – a Muslim missionary group with more than 400 members infected," *Washington Post*, April 2, 2020. https://www.washingtonpost.com/world/asia_pacific/india-coronavirus-tablighi-jamaat-delhi/2020/04/02/abd-c5af0-7386-11ea-ad9b-254ec99993bc_story.html

15. The New York Times, "Proselytizing robots': Inside South Korean Church at outbreak's center," March 10, 2020. https://www.nytimes.com/2020/03/10/world/asia/south-korea-coronavirus-shincheonji.html?action=click&module=RelatedLinks&pgtype=Article
The New York Times, "New Rochelle, once a coronavirus hot spot, may now offer hope," March 27, 2020. https://www.nytimes.com/2020/03/27/nyregion/new-rochelle-coronavirus.html
Tangi Salaün, "Special report: Five days of worship that set a virus time bomb in France," *Reuters*, March 30, 2020. https://www.google.com/amp/s/mobile.reuters.com/article/amp/idUSKBN21H0Q2

16. SITE Intelligence Group, "Recent far-right updates on the COVID-19 pandemic," May 6–12, 2020.

17. Straits Times, "London police arrest 2 teenagers linked to Covid-19 racist assault on Singaporean student," March 6, 2020. https://www.straitstimes.com/singapore/london-police-arrest-2-teenagers-linked-to-covid-19-racist-assault-on-singaporean-student

18. https://t.me/s/CoronaChanNews?before=229

19. Ibid.

20. Ibid.

21. Ibid.

22. ADL, "White supremacists respond to coronavirus with violent plots and online hate," March 26, 2020. https://www.adl.org/blog/white-supremacists-respond-to-coronavirus-with-violent-plots-and-online-hate

23. AFP, "German extremists plan May 1 protests against coronavirus restrictions," May 1, 2020. https://www.straitstimes.com/world/europe/german-extremists-plan-may-1-protests-against-coronavirus-restrictions

24. SITE Intelligence Group, "Recent far-right updates on the COVID-19 pandemic," May 13–26, 2020.

References

ADL. "White supremacists respond to coronavirus with violent plots and online hate." March 26, 2020. https://www.adl.org/blog/white-supremacists-respond-to-coronavirus-with-violent-plots-and-online-hate

———. "German extremists plan May 1 protests against coronavirus restrictions." May 1, 2020. https://www.straitstimes.com/world/europe/german-extremists-plan-may-1-protests-against-coronavirus-restrictions

DW. "Coronavirus: UK rail worker dies after 'carrier' spat on her." May 12, 2020. https://amp.dw.com/en/coronavirus-uk-rail-worker-dies-after-carrier-spat-on-her/a-53417624

Goodnough, Abby. "Prosecutors turn to Padilla for closing arguments." *The New York Times*, August 14, 2007. https://www.nytimes.com/2007/08/14/us/14padilla.html

Halpin, James, and Kalinowski, Bob. "Hanover township woman charged in Gerrity's supermarket coughing episode." *The Times-Tribune*, March 26, 2020. https://m.the-times-tribune.com/coronavirus/hanover-township-woman-charged-in-gerrity-s-supermarket-coughing-episode-1.2611519

International Crisis Group. "Contending with ISIS in the time of coronavirus." March 31, 2020. https://www.crisisgroup.org/global/contending-isis-time-coronavirus

Malaysiakini. "Yazid a member of JI Malaysia, witness tells court." October 7, 2015. https://m.malaysiakini.com/news/314941

Meek, James Gordon. "Terrorist groups spin COVID-19 as God's 'smallest soldier' attacking West." *ANC News*, April 2, 2020. https://www.google.com/amp/s/abcnews.go.com/amp/International/terrorist-groups-spin-covid-19-gods-smallest-soldier/story%3fid=69930563

Middle East Monitor. "Tunisia announces failure of a 'terrorist plot' to spread coronavirus." April 17, 2020. https://www.google.com/amp/s/www.middleeastmonitor.com/20200417-tunisia-announces-failure-of-a-terrorist-plot-to-spread-coronavirus/amp/

Naar, Ismaeel. "Coronavirus: Muslim Brotherhood activist calls on Egyptians to infect officials." *Al Arabiya English*, March 18, 2020. https://english.alarabiya.net/en/media/digital/2020/03/18/Coronavirus-Muslim-Brotherhood-activist-calls-on-Egyptians-to-infect-officials.html

NBC NEWS. "Al-Qaida takes center stage in Padilla trial." June 25, 2007. http://www.nbcnews.com/id/19420820/ns/us_news-security/t/al-qaida-takes-center-stage-padilla-trial/#.XwKcMygzaiN

Salaün, Tangi. "Special report: Five days of worship that set a virus time bomb in France." *Reuters*, March 30, 2020. https://www.google.com/amp/s/mobile.reuters.com/article/amp/idUSKBN21H0Q2

SITE Intelligence Group. "Call for violence to reopen Philippine Mosque closed by COVID-19 restrictions." May 22, 2020. https://ent.siteintelgroup.com/Jihadist-Threat-Southeast-Asia/call-for-violence-to-reopen-philippine-mosques-closed-by-covid-19-restrictions.html

———. "Recent far-right updates on the COVID-19 pandemic." May 6–12, 2020 https://theowp.org/reports/the-far-right-has-exploded-along-with-covid-19/.

Slater, Joanna, Masih, Niha, and Irfan, Shams. "India confronts its first coronavirus 'super-spreader' – a Muslim missionary group with more than 400 members infected." *Washington Post*, April 2, 2020. https://www.washingtonpost.com/world/asia_pacific/india-coronavirus-tablighi-jamaat-delhi/2020/04/02/abdc5af0-7386-11ea-ad9b-254ec99993bc_story.html

Straits Times. "London police arrest 2 teenagers linked to Covid-19 racist assault on Singaporean student." March 6, 2020. https://www.straitstimes.com/singapore/london-police-arrest-2-teenagers-linked-to-covid-19-racist-assault-on-singaporean-student

The Brussels Times. "Coronavirus: Belgium makes spitting punishable by fines and jail time." March 31, 2020. https://www.brusselstimes.com/brussels/103711/coronavirus-belgium-makes-spitting-punishable-by-fines-and-jail-time/

The New Arab. "Malaysia releases scientist who tried to build biological weapons for Bin Laden." November 21, 2019. https://english.alaraby.co.uk/english/news/2019/11/21/malaysia-releases-bin-ladens-anthrax-scientist

The New York Times. "Proselytizing robots': Inside South Korean Church at outbreak's center." March 10, 2020. https://www.nytimes.com/2020/03/10/world/asia/south-korea-coronavirus-shincheonji.html?action=click&module=RelatedLinks&pgtype=Article

———. "New Rochelle, once a coronavirus hot spot, may now offer hope." March 27, 2020. https://www.nytimes.com/2020/03/27/nyregion/new-rochelle-coronavirus.html

Terrorism Research and Analysis Consortium (TRAC). "Corona: It is the prayer of the people of al-Baghouz, whom you burned alive, it has killed you so reap the results of your actions." March 23, 2020. https://www.trackingterrorism.org/chatter/cgi-green-b1rds-unofficial-islamic-state-corona-it-prayer-people-al-baghouz-whom-you-burned-

Weaver, Matthew, and Dodd, Vikram." Coronavirus outbreak, police examine CCTV footage of suspect who spat at UK rail worker who later died." *The Guardian*, May 13, 2020. https://www.google.com/amp/s/amp.theguardian.com/world/2020/may/13/police-examine-cctv-footage-of-suspect-who-spat-at-uk-rail-worker-who-later-died

2 Decoding the global security threat of COVID-19

Mohd Mizan Aslam

Introduction

None of the nations were prepared when COVID-19 first struck the world (Ghebreyesus, 2020). It took most countries off guard as they had been in protected and comfortable zones for a significant period of time, slow to react toward the needs of extensive preparation for a pandemic (Aslam, 2020). The perils of COVID-19 indicate the flaw in the management of global security, particularly from aspects relating to defense, food safety, health, and other related sectors. The world is anticipated to be in a state of crisis if the pandemic prolongs. Although it is clear that COVID-19 has had a vast effect on the economy (Kalbana and Chan, 2020), the dangers with regard to safety and defense aspects are substantial. The absence of economic growth significantly affects the security and defense industry of a nation.

The world has often focused more on defense safety and the general safety of a nation compared to others. Ever since the Second World War approximately 70 years ago, many nations have expended hundreds of millions or a big percentage of the nation's budget to acquire military equipment such as fighter jets, ships, tanks, artillery, and bombs (Chu and Gupta, 1998). Another main target of every country, regardless of superpowers or small nations, is to claim the ownership of military technology and intelligence. In truth, there are nations that develop their own personal military technology and intelligence on the required capacity to safeguard the people and the sovereignty of the country (Hechter, 1992). All the nations worldwide are competing in advancing their technology and investing in these strategic assets.

As the world's leading arms manufacturer, United States, Russia, China, India, and England have come to be financially competent because of the sales of weapons (Kalbana and Chan, 2020) Many countries allocate a significant amount of their state provisions for military and safety, indirectly very beneficial for the growth of the world arms industry. Although a particular nation is not involved in war, having the most recent and most advanced assets in military is a representation of sovereignty and power. Large-scale weapon transactions were implemented in conflict- or war-stricken countries like the Middle East and Africa. A number of these countries are proxies for the arms race between

DOI: 10.4324/9781003197416-2

the West and the East. More than 80% of these countries will concentrate on defense and safety instead of basic living necessities like accommodation, food, and health (Davis, 2006).

At times when higher life expectancy rates are experienced by the world, most countries neglect to ensure the safety of their food and health industries. Initially, a new type of virus was identified in China, thus since December 2019 it was known as the Wuhan virus before it was widely referred to as COVID-19 from the beginning of 2020 (Pomeroy, 2020). Nevertheless, it began to show a huge impact on China at the end of January 2020, driving the government of China to enforce a full lockdown in early February 2020. At this point in time, nations started to learn about the death-threatening virus, branded as coronavirus. Subsequently, coronavirus spread to the entire world, causing the World Health Organization (WHO) to announce it as a pandemic. Consequently, the WHO officially termed the virus COVID-19 and that it had spread to approximately 200 countries in the world apart from a few island nations in the pacific such as Tonga, Niue, Kiribati, Soloman Islands, and North Korea (Rodriguez, 2020).

The effect of COVID-19 is significantly undergone by every nation, resulting in the importance of defense being no longer substantial. The world began to focus on health and food safety, in addition to the redevelopment of the economic sector (Yassin, 2020). Truly, many facets concerning COVID-19 have to be discussed. The world anticipates a distressing economic recession that will result in a number of nations becoming poor. The rate of unemployment will drastically rise, resulting in the poverty gap being enlarged. World communities will live in new-normal conditions which view air travel and cross country as unimportant, social distancing and hygiene as life priority, Working-from-home as a new alternative, online learning for schools and universities as essential, and many more. Nevertheless, this article will emphasize the impact of COVID-19 on global safety aspects (Yassin, 2020).

A minimum of eight main effects of COVID-19 on global safety have been recognized. They are breakup groups, terrorism, defense industry, cybersecurity, food security, health security, local crimes, and across crime borders. These eight aspects of safety have positive and negative impacts on every single nation in the world. For the first time, world superpowers have altered their external policies to the internal safety of their respective countries (Waxman and Wilson, 2020). Indeed, the effects of COVID-19 have resulted in considerable death rates greater than a few crucial wars in history such as the Korean and Vietnam wars (McCarthy, 2020). This evidently suggests how COVID-19 has affected the whole world, demanding them to re-assess their safety policies. Which is of paramount value in determining the safety of a nation?

Global safety essentially includes all aspects of life as well as food and health safety. This seems to be the most appropriate time to re-assess a country's vital needs and the reliance on a lot of imported products. The pandemic plainly indicates how imbalanced the world trade is. The main power blocks are perceived to take over certain sectors to ensure that globalization becomes a platform for economic growth (Aslam, 2016). China's control over the health industry has been unpleasant on the whole, particularly when China had to shut its port and stop exports for the safety of the country and its people.

A nation's level of dependence on other nations also positions the world in a state of imbalance and exposure to risks (Yassin, 2020). An identical situation is also seen in the food industry, which has led to the cut-off of food supply to the local market in some countries. The domino effect of COVID-19 has also led to online and cross-border crimes to escalate. In a wider landscape, the pandemic has also resulted in the increase of violence-related actions in some countries such as Indonesia, Nigeria, and Iraq. Nonetheless, the rate of terrorism has begun to significantly drop globally (Aslam, 2019a).

Areas of conflict

The effect on the first global security includes the movement of groups such as the separatist and rebel groups. Separatist groups that exist in countries such as Thailand, the Philippines, Azerbaijan, Bosnia, France, Georgia, Germany, Italy, Poland, and Romania are highly affected by the pandemic that is spreading (DW, 2020). The separatist movement was instantaneously halted as the death threat due to COVID-19 is ironically more daunting in comparison to death as a result of battles with the royal military. The separatist movement is weakened owing to the lack of food and supplies, alongside the restrictions on available resources. The people who have suffered and struggled to obtain basic needs in regions where conflicts have long existed are now faced with the challenges of COVID-19. Thus, they have to decide which to prioritize.

The medical systems and supplies of regions under conflict are normally inadequate; health facilities in run-down conditions as a result of war and prolonged conflicts. Moreover, the shortage of medical staff such as nurses and doctors makes it more difficult for this group. Any health assistance for the population in the areas of conflict is deemed challenging and almost impossible. Therefore, it is also one possible factor causing the spread of the COVID-19 to be worsened (GHRP, 2020). COVID-19 is expected to take a toll on women and children. In addition, domestic violence is also anticipated to rise because of the many constraints executed in these regions of conflict, such as social distancing and working from home (Koya, 2020).

Global ceasefire is essential when faced with a situation of a pandemic. Strategically, this is the best time to put away all aggressions and concentrate on establishing relationship among human beings and cooperation in dealing with COVID-19. Under the name of humanity, all shots, attacks, and bombings have to be at a standstill. The distress caused by COVID-19 should not be further burdened with the news of death due to war and conflict (Aslam, 2020). Once everything subsides, every group in conflict will need to go back to the negotiation table and resolve all related issues wisely and sincerely. The world does not want to witness some becoming victims of bombings or shootings while being treated in hospitals or while practicing social distancing.

Now is also the most suitable time for these allies to confront each other in order to deal with the problem of COVID-19. Together, the disputing parties can produce a suitable and applicable instrument to fight the virus. Their strength in asset and finance enables them to concentrate on managing matters pertaining to hospital facilities, sanitation, and prevention. The dangers of COVID-19 demand the support of every party; the achievement when facing this virus highly depends on the involvement of numerous parties and not merely on a single party.

Besides the normal routine, the emphasis on human relief should also be readdressed to aid in dealing with COVID-19. If required, many programs and activities have to be put on hold so that more room can be given to the approaches to control COVID-19. Even though the human task forces are not required to escape from the present state of affairs in refugee camps or in the regions of conflict, they are expected to improve personal safety and take steps of precaution. Planned methods of humanity programs have to be transformed into education and awareness on techniques to deal with the present pandemic situation (Samad, 2020). Those living in the areas of conflict have to be susceptible to living the right way and in new norm situations (Samad, 2020).

If observed, the Aceh Independence Movement (Gerakan Aceh Merdeka [GAM]) was effectively dismissed as a result of the tsunami disaster in the Asia-Pacific in 2004 (Aslam, 2009, 2019a). The oppositions, the GAM and the National Indonesian Army (Tentera National Indonesia [TNI]), moved their focus from war to conserving the areas seriously affected by the catastrophe. The death toll, which totaled up to hundreds of thousands in Aceh, was a massive loss to both conflicting parties. The Indonesian government, with assistance from international agencies, recreated Aceh with a socio-political landscape that is extremely different from the original situation in Aceh. The regional situation is calmer and better compared to the situation prior to the disaster.

A similar situation should be constructed if numerous contradictory parties are certain that COVID-19 is a matter that has more advantages than drawbacks. Keeping positive and pushing aside all disputes is important to shape a better life (Gunaratna et al., 2011). It is time to demonstrate to the world that humanity overrides both political and personal agendas. In order to make sure battles are ended, it is high time that the world unites and cooperates with one another. External policies set by superpower countries must be changed so that it no longer overpowers and aggravates the prevailing conflict but instead be directed to reciprocal profits leading to general sustainability and well-being.

Religious leaders are also believed to hold a vital role in evading prolonged conflict (Gunaratna, 2018). In March 2020, Pope Francis sought the countries in the world to stop the conflicts at that time. Alternatively, the world is required to encourage peace and safety, as well as to welcome diplomacy. The same issue was also expressed by Archbishop of Canterbury, Justin Welby, who required everyone to work together in handling COVID-19 regardless of religion, race, or nationality.

Africa

With regards to these calls, the unity of African countries demanded the regions of conflict in the Gambia, Sierra Leone, Togo, Costa Rica, and Niger to put down their arms. These countries are required to be at one with the other nations in the entire world while putting on spirits of humanity and stopping conflicts faced. As reported by Secretary-General of the UN dated April 2, 2020, Sudan, a country separated into two due to civil war, stated that ceasefire is implemented although only by one party, in the region of Darfur (United Nations, 2020). The Sudan Liberation Army (SLA), which is located in the region of Jebel Marra, decided on a de-facto ceasefire. Soon after, it was followed by the People's Liberation Movement-North and Sudan Revolutionary Forces (SRF). All three groups contradict but later decided to sign a peaceful ceasefire treaty organized by United Nations–African Union Mission in Darfur (UNAMID) (United Nations, 2020).

Similarly, a comparable scenario may also be observed in Cameroon. On March 25, 2020, the Southern Cameroon Defense Forces (SCDF), the armed right wing of the African People's Liberation Movement, declared a ceasefire. SCDF appealed to all Cameroon parties in conflict to discontinue the war and sit down for a discussion. Furthermore, SCDF appealed for a peace dialogue to be run on with the intention of avoiding any form of anguish that may be faced by the groups in conflict. The UN was requested to be the architect to organize the peace in Cameroon. In order for the conflict in Cameroon to end, it calls for genuine commitment from a number of parties that will consequently allow humanitarian aids to be flowed in to evade huge disasters caused by COVID-19 (United Nations, 2020).

On March 18 and 21, the treaty of the Government of Libya National Accord was sealed, declaring that it is vital to create peace with the intention to address the issue of COVID-19 in Libya and other African regions. The leader of the Libyan National Army (LNA), General Khalifa Haftar, had requested for the UN to be the arbitrator in discontinuing and subsequently resolving the country's conflict. Nevertheless, a day later, an armed battle supervened in Abu Grein, Zuwara, and Gharyan, which resulted in death and destruction (Djalloh, 2020). Comparatively, despite the awareness to put an end to the conflict while dealing with the fact that the danger of COVID-19 actually exists, the inability to realize that a larger threat awaits them is the reason the conflict continues. As a result, another treaty was signed on April 2, and to date, Libya continues to be efficacious in escaping any form of battle. It is expected that the collaboration will be sustained based on the spirit of the ceasefire treaty signed in Berlin, Germany, on January 19, 2020 (DW, 2020).

Asia

It is highly imperative that in this article the effects of COVID-19 in Asia will be examined. Afghanistan is, without doubt, the longest region of conflict in Asia. Fortunately, an agreement of understanding was sealed on February 29, 2020, between the United States and the Taliban. The agreement was made before the COVID-19 threat escalated, coercing the WHO to declare it as a pandemic. Although the agreement was not made as a result of COVID-19, it incidentally succeeded in stopping the progression of the conflict in Afghanistan. United Nations Assistance Mission in Afghanistan (UNAMA) had requested for all disputes to be stopped immediately (United Nations, 2020). The European Union Special Envoy on March 31 also commended for all conflicts to be ended to facilitate human aids to be sent to Afghanistan, immediately after COVID-19 was identified in the nation. On the contrary, the Organization of Islamic Cooperation (OIC) urged that all conflicts be ended so that peace can be established in Afghanistan (United Nations, 2020). Iran, an ally to the Taliban, also called for a ceasefire to be realized in the name of humanity.

Another region of conflict is Myanmar. In Myanmar, the areas of Rakhine and Chin are the main points of conflict, where the subject of citizens without nationalities is the Rohingya. The clash occurs between the separatist groups Arakanese Rohingya Solidarity Army (ARSA) and Tatmadaw Army which is supported by Yangoon (Hechter, 1992). Even though the UN had insisted on ceasefire in these two regions, their reactions were disappointing. The Tatmadaw Army view the treaty as idealistic and wasted effort (Gunaratna and Ali, 2014). The numerous groups concerned have to play their parts in order to stop the conflict in other regions like Kachin and Shan. The crisis in the region of Rakhine would have a negative effect if not brought to an end before COVID-19 hit Myanmar.

If this pandemic is not controlled, the lives of millions of Rohingya at refugee camps in the region of Cox Bazaar and Teknaf in Bangladesh will certainly be affected and be in extremely disadvantaged situations (Aslam, 2019a). It is a prerequisite that the conflicts formed between the government military and separatists be stopped instantaneously. Superpowers with interests in the geopolitical economy in the region of Rakhine, such as China, America, Japan, and India, must earnestly play a role in urging the ceasefire on the conflicting parties. The Rohingya refugees need humanitarian aids and, more importantly, education and awareness on how COVID-19 could be more dangerous if they breastfed among them. Challenging and underprivileged living conditions in refugee camps, along with unsystematic infrastructure and hygiene, will definitely make it the biggest humanitarian disaster lest the conflict can be stopped and all interrelated aids will be able to be transported into the regions of conflict (United Nations, 2020).

Similarly, the Philippines will also experience a very precarious situation of conflict (Gunaratna, 2015). It is highly possible for the threats of COVID-19 to become a serious matter beyond control if the conflict is not kept in order. The New People's Army (NPA), which is a wing of the Communist Party of the Philippines' armed forces, has devoted itself to delay their military activities in the Philippines. President Duterte has also conveyed that the cooperated ceasefire began from March 19 till the end of April; and will be extended based on the necessities of the parties in conflict (United Nations, 2020). The Norwegian government, which is the main planner in the initial peace treaty, should be responsible in ensuring that the conflict in the Philippines is ended.

Consequently, the dispute between Moro National Liberation Front (MNLF) and Moro Islamic Liberation Front (MILF) is an issue that can destroy the social structure and community in the Philippines (Aslam, 2020). The two separatist groups have been fighting for their own country and the autonomy by the Philippines government through the formation of Autonomous Region Muslim Mindanao (ARMM) (Aslam, 2008, 2009). Nur Misuari, in a media broadcast dated March 17, had called for conflicts to stop and hoped that the Philippines would be protected from COVID-19 threats. In this situation, Malaysia, which was portrayed as a key mediator in several series of peace negotiations prior, must take hold of the opportunity of the COVID-19 so as to generate a positive aura that can produce a new Philippines that is more orderly and calm.

Likewise, Thailand also is not spared from any sort of conflict. Separatist groups such as the Patani Liberation United Organisation (PULO) and Barisan Revolusi Nasional (BRN) are two different entities involved directly in the conflict with the Thailand government, claiming more than 7,000 lives since 2004 (Aslam, 2005). On April 3 2020, BRN announced ceasefire against any activity associated with their fight when handling COVID-19 threats. BRN affirms that the emphasis is presently on peace-making and saving the people of Southern Thailand from the pandemic. The representative of BRN also points out that the southern Thailand people are considered the main beneficiary of their plight and should be well looked after (Gunaratna, 2018).

The Kashmir conflict is one that also demands attention. The conflict, which has been happening since 1947, was generated by India and Pakistan in one region bordering both countries (United Nations, 2020). Ever since the Kashmir conflict started, more than 80,000 people have died. Many attacks and violence regularly happen within this region, particularly concerning violent attacks on the military and general community. After the government of India announced lockdown on March 25, a total of 670 COVID-19 cases have been documented (Dharvi, 2020). Until today, the contradicting parties in Kashmir have not voiced their willingness to ceasefire. In fact, tensions aggravated when India was blamed for taking advantage of the current state by arresting and detaining the Kashmir occupants practicing home quarantine and social distancing.

Europe

The fight in Europe can be focused on several main regions, for instance, Ukraine and Cyprus (Mattu, 2012). Although there are numerous separatist groups that often trigger inner conflict in some European nations, for instance, Azerbaijan, Italy, Spain, and Georgia, the aim of this discussion will be on several substantial regions facing difficulties and COVID-19 threats. From the days after the Second World War, some new nations have repudiated the rights of particular original populations, hence producing a conflict in Europe that extends until today.

On March 24, Ukraine's Foreign Minister requested the relevant parties to order a ceasefire. His pure intents were well received by separatists governing the regions of Donetsk and Luhansk in Ukraine. Consequently, the OSCE's special spokesperson who is based in Ukraine made a statement that the ceasefire, which consisted of three main parties, was being prearranged. Therefore, on March 30, the *Tripartite Agreement* was sealed between the French–German–Ukrainian governments and the two major rebel parties in the regions of Donetsk and Luhansk. Nevertheless, the conflicts persisted and heavy gunshot attacks took place between Ukraine and the group of rebel (United Nations, 2020). Nonetheless, it is hoped that there will not be any more conflicts until COVID-19 is entirely controlled.

In Europe, Cyprus is another interesting region of conflict. The conflict on this island exists between the ethnicities of Greek and Turkish. Colonization by the British Army on the Turkish Ottoman colony in 1914 has brought about a prolonged conflict between the two ethnicities. From the time when the conflict began, thousands have died, thus making the region's socio-economy and political situations very unstable. Incidentally, the COVID-19 pandemic has resulted in the UN calling for the conflicting parties in Cyprus to end the conflicts and instead concentrate on battling the spread of the virus (United Nations, 2020). Tribes identified as Greek Cypriot and Turkish Cypriot have been asked to give collaborated statements to evade battles in the upcoming future.

Middle East

The Middle Eastern continent is the most vital continent, mainly in trades concerned with the world's oil and gas industry. Ever since the end of the 19th century, the Middle East is often in conflict and unstable. The chain of wars in this region has made the battle between them to be prolonged and, therefore, too complex to be stopped (Gunaratna et al., 2011). It is perhaps most timely for this conflict to end as the world is met with the dangers of the COVID-19 pandemic. Once oil was discovered in the 1960s, the Western Asian region has been in the center of attention for, both due to its natural resources and geopolitics (Aslam, 2020). The series of wars in Iraq, Iran, Syria, and Yemen, however, would result in this area becoming more susceptible to great disaster in the future (Okuducu, 2020).

Another region that is currently in conflict is Syria. Ever since 2013, thousands have died while millions of Syrians have become refugees in Turkey, Greece, and Europe. The situation in Syria worsened when ISIS effectively formed a government by joining forces with Iraq, which is also a region. On March 24, 2020, the UN's special delegate in Syria presented a prompt for ceasefire as per resolution 2254 (2015), where all efforts to combat COVID-19 in Syria are executed. Only when ceasefire is put to force can humanitarian aids be streamed in and parties greatly affected in the country be saved. Cases of COVID-19 and related deaths have been reported in Syria, forcing The Syrian Democratic Forces (SDF) to issue a statement about the urgency for ceasefire to be implemented in Syria (DW, 2020).

On account of this appeal, the Syrian Opposition Coalition (SOC) decided to put together all the Syrian groups in conflict and freeze all military activities. Other than COVID-19, the target now is to reduce the death rate due to war. In addition, the UN's special representative agreed to move any form of aid to assist the Syrians who had been living in deprived and constrained conditions (DW, 2020). This is also perceived as a chance to practice diplomacy and convince all oppositions to sit down and resolve the situation further.

The borders between Syria and Turkey also appear to currently be the main areas of conflict. Idlib, which was overseen by America, is presently controlled by the Turkish army. Comparatively, a peace treaty was achieved on March 5, 2020 to block all forms of military activity and military aircraft attacks in the region of Idlib and the areas surrounding it. The Turkish army collaborated with SDF to avoid any form of attacks, especially on Syrian residents and Idlib (DW, 2020). Up to today, the situation is still closely controlled and the agreement has not been broken. Golan Hill, which is also disputed by Syria and Israel, is also under control (DW, 2020). UN administration in this area, through UNDOF, has thrived in constraining chaos and death to take place. Furthermore, Israel is currently focusing strongly on tackling the problem of COVID-19 in their country.

Yemen too is a new area of conflict in the Middle East. The opposing groups, Yemen and Ansar Allah governments, have decided to execute ceasefire in order to guarantee the community's peace and safety so as to permit all methods of preparation to deal with COVID-19. Fortunately, with support from the UN, the two parties agree to end all forms of attacks. Southern Transitional Council and other ethnics in Yemen, including Houthi, Hadramout Tribal Alliance, General Council of Al-Mahra and Socotra, Federal Civil State Alliance of Political Parties and Forces, and National Resistance Forces, all approve for UN to immediately hold a ceasefire (United Nations, 2020). Therefore, the intentions of this alliance are further sustained by a variety of Yemen NGOs such as Feminist Solidarity Network, Taiz Women for Life, The Abductees Mother Association, The Southern Women for Peace, and Youth Forum for Peace. A collaborated statement supporting the initiative taken by the UN has been released by the NGOs and appeals to stop wars while suggesting ways to resolve the issue of COVID-19, which has spread worldwide.

Consequently, a precarious fight was also transpired between Houthi, backed by Iran, and the government of Saudi Arabia. Behind many kinds of promises made by conflicting groups in Yemen, the missile shooting episode to Riyadh took place on March 29, 2020. The attack was effectively tackled by Saudi Arabia outside the city of Riyadh, in the region of Jizan. International media reports indicate that the attack came from Sana'a and Hudaydah in Yemen. Several parties, as well as the UN, had insisted that the attack and conflict be stopped instantly. UN had set up a special assignment identified as UNMHA, or United Nations Mission to Support the Hudaydah Agreement, founded on the agreement number S/2019/2452 by the Security Council signed on January 19, 2019, in New York. UNMHA is a strategic program initiated by UN for ceasefire in Yemen, thus evading the counter-attack from Saudi Arabia.

This arrangement is still in practice, and every party should follow it in order for the ISSUE of COVID to be dealt with successfully, particularly by the opposing parties (United Nations, 2020).

The next region of conflict is Iraq. Given that the administration of ISIS ended within the country, America manages it through a number of armed parties by proxy (Aslam, 2016). Nonetheless, once the American army admitted defeat, Iraq became very stressful and disordered. Under the guidance of Adnan al-Zurfi, the government was perceived to whole-heartedly fight against the battle that they are facing and also simultaneously aim to avoid the COVID-19 threat (Okuducu, 2020). Al-Zurfi urged the parties in conflict to put a halt to acts of violence and concentrate on the task of battling COVID-19. Furthermore, Al-Zurfi demanded the international monitoring group to come and assist in the process of ceasefire. Moqtada al-Sadr, Iraq's Syiah, also made a statement to the government of al-Zurfi on March 25 regarding the issue of ceasefire and to postpone the war until the COVID-19 pandemic is under control (Okuducu, 2020). This Iraqi situation is apparently fundamental; if this conflict can be successfully ended, so can the conflict in Yemen, Syria, and Libya, whereby each of them can be associated with one another, since there is a clear relation between them.

The subsequent war requires strict and instantaneous action with regards to the Israel-Palestine conflict. The prolonged conflict in humanitarian history began since Israel was formed as a nation on May 14, 1948 (William, 2006). One of the most prevalent concerns of this conflict is the intruding settlement of Israel on Palestine grounds. To deal with this, from time to time the Palestinians schedule violent attacks on the Israelis in order to block small and prearranged movements by Tel Aviv. Prior to the COVID-19 pandemic, a ceasefire pact took place in November 2019. The treaty was still used and should be upheld by Israel and Palestine to make sure that the conflict is not expanded (United Nations, 2020). Even though the UN established a Special Coordinator for the Middle East Peace Process (UNSCO), it is normally unsuccessful in regulating conflict that transpires between the two countries. In order to solve this, both Israel and Palestine are entailed to accept the executed ceasefire. The number of deaths among the Palestinians due to the cruelty of the Israelis is still comparatively small compared to deaths and damages after the attack of the pandemic.

Latin America

Colombia is another region of conflict that has resulted in many human losses. Although affected by a variety of criminal events, mainly drug cartels, attacks between the government and protestors have been in continuity for hundreds of years. The National Liberation Army (ELN) is perceived as a party that causes chaos in Colombia regularly (Gunaratna, 2015). The outcome of prompts from the UN and international organizations have resulted in a treaty of ceasefire to be signed between ELN and the Colombian government on April 1, 2020 (United Nations, 2020). This agreement seeks the government and protestors to follow the agreement and promote peace discourses. More remarkably, ELN further decided to deal with the danger of COVID-19 together with the government through military movements and assets owned. This announcement was well received by all parties as well as the Peace Commission of Congress, which was set up during the international initiative in Cuba in 2012 (BBC News, 2019). As the key designer of the treaty, the Norway government was also content with the treaty attained by the Colombian government and ELN. Therefore, all attacks were halted and COVID-19 was made the main focus.

A similar situation is believed to hit a few nations in other Latin American regions including Venezuela. As Hugo Chavez and Nicholas Maduro contest for the president seat, Venezuela is brought into a conflict and a civil war was nearly struck (BBC News, 2019). The power struggle has resulted in an increased mortality rate, anarchy, and damage, which, in due course, has caused the government of Venezuela big concern. Hugo Chavez openly announced in Caracas that the opponents made an arrangement with an outsider centered in Florida to aid the process of dethroning President Nicholas Maduro. While the entire world was fighting to overcome the COVID-19 pandemic, Venezuela was on the verge of civil war (United Nations, 2020). After thousands became infected with COVID-19 in Venezuela, it is time to concentrate on the ceasefire and thrive on the collaboration between the government and the opposition so as to eradicate COVID-19. The same condition is also believed to be happening in Peru, as part of the group loyal to ex-president Alberto Fujimori and the current leader, Pedro Pablo Kuczynski (DW, 2020).

Terrorism activities

Significantly, all terrorism activities in the world were stopped instantly. ISIS and Al-Qaeda movements are believed to focus more on finding solutions to the COVID-19 pandemic compared to launching attacks and bombs. Initially, terrorist activities were intended to put together a nation based on an Islamic dynasty centered in particular regions including Iraq and Syria (Djalloh, 2020). The arrival of the COVID-19 virus was first regarded as god's army sent to destroy enemies of Islam such as America, England, and China. Nevertheless, when COVID-19 began to attack the entire world as well as Muslim countries, their views were altered. Offensive narratives aimed toward nations categorized as non-believers disappeared all of a sudden.

However, during the COVID-19 pandemic, we still hear of terrorism attacks taking place in a few nations in the world. One of them occurred in Indonesia on April 17, 2020. The Syariah Mandiri bank robbery was executed by a group of terrorists in Kabupaten Poso, Sulawesi, with the excuse of Fai' (Stanislaus et al., 2020). One of the attackers was shot by the Indonesian Police. The attackers, Ali Darwin aka Gobel, and Muis Fahron aka Abdullah, both members of East Mujahidin Indonesia (MIT), were shot by the Indonesian Police (POLRI) after they threw a Molotov cocktail. In Medan, a bomb was detonated on March 25, 2020, causing three people to die. The explosion at the Ramayana restaurant was aimed at the Hindus during the Nyepi celebration organized by the followers of Jamaat Ansarut Daulah (JAD) (Stanislaus. et al., 2020). On April 25, 2020, three terrorists were arrested in relation to the terrorist attacks in Makassar.

The following case happened in London on April 13. Sudesh Amman committed a violent attack by stabbing another man aged 40 years old and a female motorcycle rider aged 50 in the city of London (Simone, 2020). The man was thought to act in the name of religion and called for a pledge of obedience (baia'h) to ISIS. Sudesh was shot at Streatham High Road while wearing a bulletproof vest. A month before the incident, a terrorist attack also took place close to London Bridge and ended with two injured and the attacker dead. Several other terrorist incidents were also reported in England during the COVID-19 period of.

Similarly, Africa also faced terrorist attacks on large scales, although pressured with COVID-19. Boko Haram in Nigeria was alleged to start attacking areas of Lake Chad Basin, resulting in 92 deaths (Djalloh, 2020). Johns Hopkins University states in its latest report dated April 28 that in the first few months of the COVID-19 pandemic, cases of terrorist attacks increased from 1,000 to 8,000 cases in the whole of Africa. It is also thought that members of Al-Qaeda cooperated with ISIS to perform a variety of attacks that destroyed buildings and lives in the majority of nations within the regions in African. On May 10, 2020, a suicidal bomb attack went off in Cameroon, causing 23 people to be killed. Boko Haram also teamed up with the Islamic State for West Africa Province (ISWAP), which resulted in the death of 47 Nigerian soldiers on March 24 in Yorgi, Yobe, and Nigeria (Djalloh, 2020).

On May 4, 2020, an attack targeted at the paramilitary troupe of Iraq led to 10 deaths. Abu Bakr Djalloh reports that the DW safety analyzer indicated that the attack on Iraq by ISIS is continued despite the threats of COVID-19 in the world today (Djalloh, 2020; DW, 2020). In fact, ISIS believes that COVID-19 is a small military force sent by god to eradicate all the enemies of Islam in the world. War attacks during the final week of April, i.e. the beginning of Ramadhan, killed three safety guards, while on April 29, 2020, 32 Syrian armies were killed by the suicidal attack squad in Kirkuk, Iraq (Okuducu, 2020). This clearly proves that it is difficult to put a stop to terrorist attacks in Iraq.

Even though there is a decline in the number of terrorist attacks worldwide, it is not yet substantial to indicate that terrorist decisions were affected by the COVID-19 threat (Aslam, 2020). As previously discussed, terrorists think that COVID-19 is assistance from god and a chance to perform jihad, as encouraged in Islam. Although there is a minimum drop, there is no official declaration by the higher ISIS leaders to accomplish a ceasefire order or postpone their attacks. Regardless of it being the holy month of Ramadhan, their spirits to continue their fight to form an Islamic state (daulah Islamiyyah) are not dampened.

According to the DW media report, ISIS is generating a more profitable income through black market trades, particularly petrol, antique or ancient items, and taxes (DW, 2020). Limitations and transfers to many sectors, together with transportation, offer ISIS a well-paid revenue. Moreover, the inefficient border protection of some nations has encouraged the activities of smuggling by ISIS and other criminal agencies. ISIS was stated as receiving an income of up to thousands of millions of dollars from such trades.

The safety of the food industry

Some countries that largely depend on the huge amount of imported food face a big threat. Indeed, even available food in the market may be controlled by a group with its own personal plan (Kementerian Pertahanan, 2020). The food in the market is highly exposed to threats such as being of low grade, not halal, and poisonous. The entry of imported food during critical times such as this should also be questioned in terms of safety, hygiene, and halalness. The subsequent factor is the instrument and manner the food is distributed to the target group, both demanding careful consideration. With the aim of solving all these issues, studies regarding food safety must be established if the world wishes to be free from COVID-19 and make sure that we thrive in combatting the pandemic (Kementerian Pertahanan, 2020).

The notion of safety is not just about defending the interest of the country's citizens from external dangers of enemies, but it also includes social and economic wellness protection. On the contrary, food safety is a term applied in political science which means a protection in the form of sufficient amount of food and the safety of the food content for the community (Daud et.al., 2020). It aims to protect the people from being deprived of the most rudimentary necessities, which is food (Daud 2020). Furthermore, it hopes to strengthen the efforts of agencies concerned in areas of health safety and nutrition so that national coherence can be improved in view of the needs for an integrated approach while reducing the overlapping of responsibilities that can possibly enhance the current source of expertise in both the private and public sectors (Kementerian Kewangan, 2020).

The establishment of a food safety regulatory body is essential to ascertain that general public health is guaranteed through the strengthening of food safety issues at every level of the food chain and making sure that the people achieve the level of optimum nutrition. For instance, Malaysia's imported processed food was valued at RM20 billion in 2018, a seemingly high figure for a nation with a population of only 32 million people (Mohd Shafie, 2014), implying that Malaysia relies so much on import products as food provisions for its citizens (Kementerian Pertanian, 2020). This means that food safety for the citizens is not guaranteed, although Malaysia's rank in the Global Food Safety Index (GFSI) went up to the 28th position in 2019, compared to the 48th position the year before (Samad, 2020).

According to a study conducted by (Akmal, Zahrul, Bin Damin., 2016) on the subject of agriculture-based food security, it was found the government of a nation often puts pressure in determining that the food production is stable. Such emphasis is also made by making sure that there is access to the food on a domestic level. To achieve this objective, the government has to focus on the progression policy of the food agriculture, although faced with three main challenges: change of government focus from an agricultural country to industrial, dependence on imported food, and climate change that can disrupt food safety.

A variety of studies with regards to food safety, which were carried out before this, focused more on the spread of other epidemics such as H1N1 (Mohd Ali, 2008; Mat, Othman, & Mohd Kamal, 2018) and SARS (Mohd Shafie, 2014; Shamsudin, 2016). A study conducted by looks at the effectiveness of food management during a natural disaster. Food safety only centers on demand and offer in a situational crisis, as initially stated (Kementerian Kewangan, 2020). Most existing research emphasizes food needs instead of food safety.

Nevertheless, research regarding food safety conducted during the spread of the COVID-19 virus is very restricted. Furthermore, it is on average the first time for all the people and nations in the world to handle the subject of COVID-19 without explicitly given guidelines, particularly in handling safety and food management in a lockdown situation. Sity Daud (2020) pointed out that food safety is widely practiced in Europe as a non-urgent technique which is more of an awareness process instigated by NGOs and charity bodies. However, food safety is vital in a lot of countries dealing with the threat of the COVID-19 pandemic.

With respect to this, all the nations worldwide are required to develop their Food Safety Policy that can be applied during any crisis or during the COVID-19 pandemic. Most nations have not yet developed a distinct policy on food safety that can be referred to when facing an epidemic or pandemic. Literature shows that only China and Belgium have designed a comprehensive policy on food safety controls during the spread of the COVID-19 pandemic (Suhor et al., 2014; Akmal, 2016). Fundamentally, the structure of the food safety policy is imperative so that the process of assessing the level of a nation's preparation to face a crisis as immense as this is eased (Aslam, 2019a). The main function of food safety is to help the government effectively survive in such a situation or when hit with a crisis.

Safety of the health industry

The COVID-19 pandemic clearly portrays the level of world dependence on health products produced in China. The world is now aware that 60–80% of pharmaceutical medication production originates from China (Samad, 2020). In truth, even America discloses that antibiotics, ibuprofen, Vitamin C, and many other basic medicines are also imported from China. Yanzhong Huang, senior fellow for global health at the Council on Foreign Relations of the United States acknowledges that 90% of the medicines in Uncle Sam's market originates from China (Samad, 2020).

The world cannot refute China's ability to produce numerous pharmaceutical items on the capacity of mass production and low-cost manpower (Veena, 2020). China also has many industrial plantations that can produce all sorts of medication or pharmaceutical facilities needed by the world. China is capable of manufacturing millions of medicines, if necessary. Additionally, cheap and keen labor devoted to work has made China a giant medical industry. Subsequently is technology. China has prospered in developing various kinds of technologies that can quicken the process of producing a certain product and in large quantities.

The enhancement of globalization also demands the world to change its attention on the production of certain products at reduced cost rates. Thus, this is why all types of companies, including those from the West, have started to shut their factories in western countries and other locations. They concentrate on setting up production in China as it is cheaper, and several support services and incentive programs are also provided by the Chinese government (Samad, 2020). It is therefore not a surprise if even Steve Jobs opened a plant producing iPhones in China and later marketed them in the United States. The same applies to other big names in the trade including luxury items such as watches and women's handbags which are also produced in China and go through detailed control yet are efficient in terms of production costs.

China is not required to wait for copyright process patents that often take a long waiting period, as practiced in the West (Aslam, 2019a). Instead, China will immediately work on certification processes and other related procedures. Indirectly, this enhances the industry in China, particularly those focused on medication. Pharmaceutical equipment from huge machines to small masks are also produced by China in large amounts, ranging from cheap to more sophisticated designs, as a result of R&D and mass production (Aslam, 2005).

Since rules associated with environmental pollution are very unprofessionally managed in China, it therefore indirectly becomes an advantage to industrial players related to medicine. If compared to Europe and other advanced nations, the law and rigid regulations have become a bit of a hindrance in the nation's industrial development with reference to medicine (William, 2006). Human rights groups, *green-peace* movements and law practitioners will always look for means to prevent various activities believed to be unethical or against any human rights. Nonetheless, this state does not occur in China, whereby industries are permitted to carry out whatever activity they desire as long as they give good returns to the citizens and country (Samad, 2020).

The Chinese government is also known to offer attractive subsidies to industrial players so that they are involved in a cost-effective business. The Chinese government encourages all kinds of industries and supplies the required form of aid needed. Every district in China has its own industry that progresses very quickly (Samad, 2020). The construction of new industrial regions in numerous districts makes China a production center of various products, especially health-related products. The roads that link China with all states and ports are also the fundamental reason for China's industrial strength.

The world does not seem to realize the high level of dependency on China, to the extent that no one has considered building their own health industry. The broad opening of the capitalist economic market and globalization has resulted in opportunities for trade to develop. The supply and demand model has transformed China into a world trading center. Each nation is searching for efficiently produced items sold at a low cost (Aslam, 2005). The middle man is often anticipating the chance to generate money through import and export activities. Hence, incidentally, China is a country where all types of medicine needed by different parties can be obtained. It is also thought that crime and corruption both play a role in the industry until it is well sheltered and promptly grown without any obstacles (Aslam, 2020).

Today, China is advancing with the application of the 5G technology. Similarly, goods production uses a far more advanced technology compared to the West. Thus China is perceived as a superpower in the health industry (Samad, 2020). With the event of the COVID-19 pandemic, the world needs to witness all this. No matter how or in whatever situation, every country in the world should have an industry associated with health. The safety of the health industry is very important, specifically in times of crisis, as is presently happening. Once a pandemic starts all countries will protect and complete the requirements of their own people. Ports, as well as air, sea, and ground route closures, will cause the state during a pandemic to be critical. At this point, a country must be able to meet its domestic needs, especially health products and medication. Basic industries such as face masks, surgical masks, and hand sanitizers are essential and need to be possessed by every country (Aslam, 2020).

Other than this, the management of good health in relation to the distribution of medication and medical equipment is also vital. Every nation not only needs a health industry, but they also have to regulate and manage it during times of crisis. COVID-19 clearly shows that national front liners are the medical teams and not the security team or teams with advanced defense weapons (Aslam, 2020). Many countries are short of the advanced military force or volume but are regarded great because they can effectively control the threat of COVID-19. This is an indication of how these countries manage to constrain the attack of COVID-19 well and orderly.

Criminal activities across borders

Crime is one of the other impacts of COVID-19. Various local and international crimes have been reported during the spread of this pandemic. Stakeholders often search for space and opportunity to maneuver the COVID-19 situation to gain profit. Although generally, the drop in crime rates is detailed, the virus is still mutating. Criminals will often be more advanced in their activities than us (Special Branch, 2020).

In Brazil and England, it has been recorded that drugs have been delivered using drones. Numerous drug consumptions and wild parties are organized privately by using many types of applications that may be downloaded on smartphones. Somehow, prostitution activities still continue with the use of delivery services and many more. Even syndicates of online gambling, pornography, online scams and others, intend to expand during the COVID-19 season (Special Branch, 2020). This evidently shows that threat to security still takes place although COVID-19 is spread within a country and among its nationals. A number of countries have authorized access to the internet in order to fill up the boredom of staying at home. Even though many use this facility for educational activities and additional knowledge, there are also those who abuse the pre-determined facilities. A number of reports also illustrate how online scams are rapidly spread. Many are misled with all sorts of fake websites and applications created. Every new product created by the government will surely be created on fake websites to confuse people, just like it happens in Malaysia, Thailand, Indonesia, Brazil, and America. Communities who spend a lot of time on the computer or use the internet are powerful targets of this group of scammers.

Cross-border crimes are also extensively documented during the COVID-19 season. Various crimes related to illegal immigrants, drug smuggling (contraband), firearms, human trafficking, and many more are recorded during COVID-19 (Aslam, 2020). Countries such as Greece, Cyprus, England, Malaysia, and Australia, which are often targets of immigrants, continue to display an increase in illegal immigrants. These criminals do not fear the virus but they are more particular about profits from hidden luxurious businesses which do not demand a big capital. It is a modern form of slavery that happens in many areas of the world today. This syndicate portrays good space and opportunity as a result of restricted observation in the borders and entrance of a country.

Besides this, the entry of an immigrant or illegal immigrant is also thought to have a security impact if they bring in the virus with them. They actually have high potentials in bringing COVID-19 or whatever virus to the countries entered. The virus will spread among them and consequently to the general public they are in physical contact with. Eventually, a country's safety is put in jeopardy and thus exposed to socio and economic annihilation.

Successively, the security threat at the times of COVID-19 is associated with the spread of false news. Many countries have to tighten their law or create a new act to hinder the spread of false news and information, especially with regards to COVID-19 (Kementerian Pertahanan, 2020). All sorts of false information spread in a lot of countries have resulted in panic among the people. The government is forced to mobilize the army, police, and certain assets in order to control the instability that occurs. It is therefore essential for a country to form a precise set of rules to stop the spread of false news and outrun the group better known as "the keyboard warrior," which is a group looking for publicity from others' difficulties (Aslam, 2019b).

Criminal threat as a result of COVID-19 is also associated with hackers. This group of hackers sees the whole world migrating from a conventional system to the internet or an online-based system. The use of many open-source platforms has put the security data system of a certain agency or country into a risky position. There are government agencies that use open stages because they lack preparation to face the COVID-19 threat. As a result, some agencies were attacked and their data platforms were hacked. This situation will be more unsafe if private information leaks and falls into the hands of the enemy or certain parties that will make it as "ransomware" (Aslam, 2019b).

Conclusion

The world is now in a huge crisis. After the Second World War ended, most countries in the world have been in their comfort zones and have not prepared to face threats like this. The spread of COVID-19, which was then announced as a pandemic by the WHO, startled the world and is in search of the best remedy to tackle the situation. Every group that disputes have to return to the discussion table and agree to act in order to end the present conflict.

Every nation has to work together and those in conflict must build good collaboration among each other so that the conflict can be put to a stop. Regions under conflict such as the Middle East and South Asia, along with Latin America, are associated with other countries. The conflict demands cooperation between governments in order to end it. The success of handling a crisis will not materialize with the effort of only one party; it requires the involvement of some sincere and committed parties. It is not crucial to have hidden agendas when handling conflicts at this time, because a bigger effect concerning COVID-19 has to be thought out.

Cooperation from all sorts of Non-Governmental Agencies (NGOs) and also Civil Society Organizations (CSOs) is vital and can be moved now. Initiatives of country-community and government-private, such as in Yemen and Asia, too, seem to be a noble effort (Kruglanski et al., 2019). At present, the attainment of handling COVID-19 is not solely the responsibility of a particular country or government. It, however, appears as a collective step by involving several agencies as well as NGOs and CSOs, which have identical objectives, which are to end the disputes and consequently overcome the COVID-19 threat. Every party, including influential individuals from religious groups, women and the local leaders can also be motivated in order to end all forms of conflict in the world today.

The UN, as the uppermost body that connects all the nations in the world, must take on a more effective role. Creating a monitoring team or a group of special representatives is not adequate; in fact a more systematic and integrated movement is required to handle the conflicts that occur in the whole world. UN must encourage cooperation between all parties by firming up their understanding and avoiding prolonged conflict. The UN has to also see the issue of conflict from the perspectives of humanity and justice and not in the interest of certain parties. Is the restriction on nations such as Iran, Cuba, Libya, Sudan, and North Korea still relevant today? Do all these constraints make it more difficult for the countries to handle the spread of COVID-19? UN has to go through the steps taken and should be able to take unparalleled action with superpowers who have personal agendas. This is where the UN will be seen as a free body that fights for the fate of all the nations in the world fairly.

A brave role can also be taken by blocks of other countries such as the European Union (EU), Non-Aligned Movement (NAM), ASEAN, OECD, and others, in playing only a part in assisting the development of safety and to stop other conflicts. These countries also need to help in the process of handling COVID-19 especially through related research findings. The process of healing and using certain antidotes must also be shared among the different countries in the world. The success in handling COVID-19 is not confined to one country. If a country is free from COVID-19, but other countries still struggle to handle it, then the condition will not recover as usual. Economic, trade, and tourism activities are still affected by the pandemic phenomenon.

The COVID-19 pandemic has made it challenging to call together conflict parties in direct negotiations. It will not deter the whole world from pursuing best conflict solutions. We must be creative and use the latest technology such as IoT and Big Data to the maximum extent possible to maintain channels of communications and de-escalate conflict. This initiative needs to be backed by pro-active diplomatic engagements and actions. It is challenging to bring the voices of other actors including NGOs, CSOs, religious leaders, women, youths, and individuals in our efforts to secure sustainable agreements to uphold international peace and security.

References

Akmal, Zahrul, Bin Damin. (2016). Dasar Kerajaan dan Isu Makanan di Malaysia. Tesis PhD. Sintok: Perpustakaan UUM.

Aslam, M. M. (2005). Asian and globalization: An analysis from Tun Mahathir's perspectives. Paper presented at the International Conference of Asian Scholars. Shanghai.

Aslam, M. M. (2008). Operational and Ideological Challenges in Islamic Militancy in Malaysia: The case of Kumpulan Militan Malaysia (KMM). In Md Yatim Othman (Ed.), Malaysia in Various Issues: A Collection of Essays. New Zealand: Victoria University of Wellington.

Aslam, M. M., (2009). A Critical Study of Kumpulan Militant Malaysia, its wider connections in the region and the implications of radical Islam for the stability of South East Asia. (PhD Thesis), Victoria University of Wellington, New Zealand.

Aslam, M. M. (2016). Drugs and Cross Border Terrorism. Keynote paper presented at the 1st International Joint Conference on Drugs, Social Sciences and Technology (DRUGSTECH), 30–31 October 2016. Universitas Ubudiyah Indonesia, Banda Aceh, Indonesia.

Aslam, M. M. (2019a). Cross Border Terrorism in Terrorist Rehabilitation and Community Engagement di Malaysia and Southeast Asia. London: Routledge.

Aslam, M. M. (2019b). Artificial Intelligence (AI) Belum Cukup Bagus. Special Column in Harian Metro, June 13 2019. Kuala Lumpur: Media Prima.

Aslam, M. M. (2020). Pemahaman Agama Ketika Wabak. Terbitan Malaysiakini pada 11 April 2020. Dilayari pada 11 April 2020 di laman sesawang: https://www.malaysiakini.com/columns/520063

BBC News. (2019). Venezuela Crisis: Maduro Warns of Civil War. Retrieved on May 03 2020 from: https://www.bbc.com/news/world-latin-america-47112284

Chu, K. Y. and Gupta, S. (1998). Social Safety Nets: Issues and Recent Experiences. Washington, DC: IMF.

Daud, Sity. (2020). Dasar Pembangunan dan Populisme di Malaysia. Bangi: Penerbit UKM.

Daud, Sity, et.al. (2020). Pelan Tindakan Majlis Tindakan Kos Sara Hidup Negara, 2019–2022. Putrajaya: KPDNHEP.

Dharvi, V. (2020). Covid-19 Crisis Prolongs Kashmir Lockdown. Retrieved on April 13 2020 from: https://www.dw.com/en/covid-19-crisis-prolongs-kashmir-lockdown/a-53088317

Djalloh, Abu Bakar. (2020). Increased Terror Attacks in Africa amid Coronavirus Pandemic. Retrieved on April 10 2020 from: https://www.dw.com/en/increased-terror-attacks-in-africa-amid-coronavirus-pandemic/a-53066398

DW. (2020). IS Takes Advantage of Coronavirus to Ramp Up Attacks in Iraq & Syria. Retrieved on May 06 2020 from: https://www.dw.com/en/is-takes-advantage-of-coronavirus-to-ramp-up-attacks-in-iraq-syria/a-53321781

Ghebreyesus, T. A. (2020, April 13). WHO Director-General's Opening Remark at the Media Briefing of COVID-19 – April 13 2020. Retrieved on 3rd May 2020 from: https://www.who.int/dg/speeches/detail/who-director-general-s-opening-remarks-at-the-media-briefing-on-covid-19–13-april-2020.

Global Humanitarian Response Plan (GHRP) (April–December 2020). United Nations Coordinated Appeal April–December 2020. Retrieved on 17th of January 2021 from: https://reliefweb.int/report/world/global-humanitarian-response-plan-covid-19-april-december-2020-ghrp-july-update-enar

Gunaratna, G., Jerard J., and Rubin, L., (2011). Terrorist Rehabilitation and Counter-Radicalisation. London: Routledge.

Gunaratna, R. (2015). "Global threat assessment: A new threat on the horizon?," Counter Terrorist Trend and Analysis, A Journal of International Centre for Political Violence and Terrorism Research, S. Rajaratnam School of International Studies, vol. 7, issue 1, p. 5.

Gunaratna, R. (2018). "Counterterrorism: ASEAN Militaries' Growing Role – Analysis." RSIS Commentaries. March 14. Retrieved on June 01, 2018 from: https://www.research-gate.net/profile/Rohan-Gunaratna/publication/328530810_Counterterrorism_ASEAN_Militaries'_Growing_Role/links/5bd2d1b3299bf1124fa39d5d/Counterterrorism-ASEAN-Militaries-Growing-Role.pdf

Gunaratna, R., and Ali, M. (2014). Terrorist Rehabilitation: A New Frontier in Counter-Terrorism. London: Imperial College Press.

Hechter, M. (1992). The dynamics of secession. Acta Sociologica. vol. 35, issue 4, pp. 267–283. New York: Sage Publication Ltd.

Idris Okuducu. (2020). DAESH/ISIS Increases Attacks in Iraq Amid Virus. Retrieved on May 11 2020 from: https://www.aa.com.tr/en/middle-east/daesh-isis-increases-attacks-in-iraq-amid-virus/1832517

Interview with Perlis Special Branch Director, Royal Malaysia Police in Kangar, May 06, 2020.

Kalbana, P., and Chan, D. (2020, 2 Mei). A Longer Wait Could Have Resulted in More Losses in Revenue. Retrieved on May 03 2020 from: New Straits Times: https://www.nst.com.my/news/nation/2020/05/589227/longer-wait-could-have-resulted-more-losses-revenue pada 2 Mei 2020

Kementerian Kesihatan Malaysia. (2020). Malaysia Memulakan Kajiselidik Solidariti Global. Retrieved on April 15 2020 from: http://www.moh.gov.my/index.php/database_stores/store_view_page/21/1425

Kementerian Kewangan. (2020). Laporan Laksana Ketiga: Pelaksanaan Pakej Prihatin Rakyat. Dilayari pada April 25 2020 dari laman sesawang: https://www.treasury.gov.my/pdf/Teks-Ucapan-Laporan-LAKSANA-PRIHATIN-Ketiga.pdf

Kementerian Pertahanan. (2020). Kekang PATI, Keselamatan Negara Terus Diperketat, Kawal Pendatang. Dilayari pada April 27 2020 dari laman sesawang: http://www.mod.gov.my/ms/mediamenu/berita/701-kekang-pati-kawalan-sempadan-negara-terus-diperketat-diperhebat

Kementerian Pertanian. (2020b). Bekalan Makanan Negara Mencukupi. Dilayari pada April 13 2020 dari laman sesawang: https://www.moa.gov.my/documents/20182/197571/Bekalan+Makanan+Negara+Konsisten+dan+Mencukupi.pdf/78833140-e787-4751-8b21-586cfef7f5e8

Koya, Zakiah. (2020, 2 Mei). Be Prepared to Live with COVID-19 for the Next Two Years, Says Dr Jemilah. Diakses daripada laman web. The Star: https://thestar.com.my/news/nation/2020/05/02/be-prepared-to-live-with-covid-19-for-the-next-two-years-says-dr-jemilah pada 2 Mei 2020

Kruglanski, A., Belanger, J., and Gunaratna, R. (2019). Three Pillars of Radicalization: Needs, Narratives & Networks. Oxford: Oxford University Press.

Mat, Bakri, Othman, Zarina & Omar, Mohd Kamal. (2018). Anjakan Paradigma dalam Kajian Keselamatan Insan di Asia Tenggara. Akademika, vol. 88, issue 1, April 2018, 193–207.

Mattu, Katjuscia. (2012). Internal Colonialism in Western Europe: The Case of Sardinia. Barcelona: University of Barcelona Press.

McCarthy, N. (2020). Covid-19 Death Toll Surpasses Vietnam War. Retrieved on May 01 2020 from: https://www.statista.com/chart/21545/deaths-from-the-coronavirus-and-vietnam-war/

Mohd Ali, Khairul Anuar. (2008). Aspek Kualiti, Keselamatan Dan Kesihatan di Kalangan PKS Makanan: Satu Sorotan Kajian, Jurnal Teknologi, vol. 49, issue 1, pp. 65–69.

Mohd Shafie, Nurul Syuhada. (2014). Kajian tahap penilaian amalan keselamatan makanan di premis makanan sekitar alam mesra Kota Kinabalu. Universiti Malaysia Sabah. http://eprints.ums.edu.my/14674/(Unpublished).

Pomeroy, Ross. (2020). Why Do New Disease Outbreak Always Seems To Starts in China? Retrieved on April 12 2020 from: https://www.realclearscience.com/blog/2020/02/18/why_do_new_disease_outbreaks_always_seem_to_start_in_china.html

Rodriguez, Adriana. (2020). These Countries Have No Reports on Coronavirus Cases. But Can They Be Trusted? Retrieved on May 07 2020 from: https://www.usatoday.com/story/news/world/2020/05/06/covid-19-which-countries-have-no-coronavirus-cases/3076741001/

Samad, Joe. (2020). Covid-19: The New National Security Threat. Retrieved on April 01 2020 from: https://www.freemalaysiatoday.com/category/opinion/2020/03/31/covid-19-the-new-national-security-threat/

Shamsudin, Mad Nasir. (2016). Urban Agriculture: A Way Forward to Food and Nutrition Security in Malaysia. Procedia – Social and Behavioral Sciences, vol. 2016·January. pp. 39–45.

Simone, Daniel De. (2020). Sudesh Amman: Who Was the Streatham Attacker. Retrieved on March 03 2020 from: https://www.bbc.com/news/uk-51351885

Suhor, Shamsudin, Yusof, Sakinah S. A., Ismail, Rahmah, Aziz, Azimon Abdul, and Katini Aboo, Muhammad Rizal Razman and Talib@Khalid. 2014. Kesihatan dan Keselamatan Makanan: Kesedaran Pengguna dan Peruntukan Perundangan Kanun. Jurnal Kanun. Bangi: Penerbit UKM. Disember 2014. pp. 236–253.

Stanislaus, R., Amy, Y. S., and Benny J. M. (2020). Collaborative Governance in Terrorist Rehabilitation Program in Indonesia. Concept Paper for book proposal by Aslam, M. M. and Gunaratna, R.

Tamburino, L., Bravo, G., Clough, Y and Nicholas, K. A. (2020). From Population to Production: 50 Years of Scientific Literature on How to Feed the World. Elsevier ScienceDirect. Vol. 24: March 2020. https://www.sciencedirect.com/science/article/pii/S2211912419301798.

United Nations. (2020). Update on the Secretary General's Appeal for Global Ceasefire. Retrieved on April 10 2020 from:file:///Users/mariyani/Downloads/Update%20on%20SG%20Appeal%20for%20Ceasefire,%20April%202020%20(2).pdf

Veena, B. (2020, 2 Mei). Do It in Stages, Say Health Expert. Diakses daripada laman web. New Straits Times: https://www.nst.com.my/news/nation/2020/05/589215/do-it-stages-say-health-expert pada 2 Mei 2020.

Waxman, O. and Wilson, C. (2020). How the Coronavirus Death Toll Compares to Other Deadly Events from American History. Retrieved on April 30 2020 from: https://time.com/5815367/coronavirus-deaths-comparison/

William, C. Davis. (2006). Lone Star Rising. Texas: A&M University Press.

Yassin, Muhyiddin Mohd. (2020, 1 Mei). *Teks Perutusan Khas YAB Tan Sri Dato' Haji Muhyiddin bin Haji Mohd Yassin, Perdana Menteri Malaysia sempena Hari Pekerja.* Putrajaya: Pejabat Perdana Menteri.

3 COVID-19 crisis

The impact of trade and economic contagion on developing and emerging markets

Nihal Pitigala[1]

Introduction

The ongoing novel coronavirus (COVID-19) pandemic poses an unprecedented challenge to public health on a global scale, with cases now confirmed in more than 210 countries by the end of April 2020. As governments are scrambling to safeguard people's health, the contagion has fast extended to the economic sphere, creating an international economic crisis. Just as COVID-19 is unparalleled in our lifetime, in terms of its contagion rate and the toll on human lives, it is likewise unique in the expected economic contagion that is fundamentally different from previous shocks, such as the global financial crisis of 2008–2009 and the Great Depression.

Previous economic crises manifested either as demand shocks with one epicenter, such as the United States during the global financial crisis and the Great Depression or as supply shock, such as the 1970s OPEC oil embargo. Other localized mini-shocks such as the 2011 earthquake and tsunami in Japan triggered a supply shock that disrupted global value chains (GVCs), particularly the automotive, computer, and consumer electronics producers that rely heavily on Japanese suppliers of specialized parts and components.COVID-19, in contrast, has unleashed simultaneous global demand and supply shocks, span across all nodes and centers of economic activity across the world. The domestic economic crises are, however, not confined nor treatable within national borders. Consumers and businesses worldwide will most likely continue to practice safety measures of some form or another, even when containment measures are relaxed. With the global economy interconnected more than ever, the rate of cross-economic contagion is likely to take an unparalleled economic toll including on human capital development.

Despite massive stimulus packages being crafted as economic lifelines in some developed economies, global income this year is likely to shrink dramatically, with significant transmission effects to developing and emerging markets. The vulnerability of developing countries to the pandemic is particularly acute, with limited capacity to weather the immediate health crisis and expected economic fallout due to high pre-existing poverty rates, larger informal sectors, shallower financial markets, and less fiscal space to broaden the social safety net or to

DOI: 10.4324/9781003197416-3

stimulate their domestic economies. A protracted global depression threatens a deeply disruptive and lasting structural impact on their economies. The resulting risks pose a threat to social stability and security, particularly in countries already vulnerable pre-pandemic.

In this paper the focus is the transmission channels of COVID-19 economic contagion that adversely affect developing and emerging countries with particular reference to Sri Lanka and drawing on the lessons learned from past crises. The trade-related transmission mechanisms unveil a mix of policy levers that may shorten the depth and duration of the unfolding economic downturn and the impact on developing and emerging economies like Sri Lanka and its citizens. To mitigate the adverse impacts and adjust to the "new normal" require a potent structural element on how to trade, financial, services sector markets and efficiencies are addressed.

The unusual and highly disruptive global economic impact of COVID-19

What makes the COVID-19 health and economic crisis different from other pandemics and economic crises? First, it is a massive and highly contagious global health shock. COVID-19 combines two marked differentiators – the rates of contagion and resulting mortality. COVID-19 is proving to be far more contagious than the seasonal flu, while recent data (Johns Hopkins University & Medicine, 2020) (as of May 9, 2020) put the average global fatality rate at close to 7% and reaching above 14% in Italy, Spain, and Belgium – far higher than the 0.1% average annual fatality rate for the seasonal flu (World Health Organization, 2020). The unusual – and still not fully understood – nature of this pandemic, combined with the high degree of global connectedness, has enabled it to rapidly spread across the borders. It is likely that most, if not all countries, will be hit by the pandemic, with direct costs to their economies related to morbidity, health care, and uncertainty.

The extreme mitigation measures to contain COVID-19 have, in turn, generated sudden and dramatic reductions in domestic and external supply and demand for both goods and services, constricting the flow of goods and people. Economic contagion is now spreading as fast as the disease itself.

Those countries and regions at the center of the health and economic crises – China, the United States, and the European Union (EU) – are much more interconnected between themselves and with the rest of the world through the exchange of goods, services, financial, and people-to-people interactions. Within countries, the virus has hit primarily large, internationally integrated production and service centers (e.g. Wuhan, Daegu, Milan, Munich, Seattle, New York). The scale and uncertain trajectory of the infection are also reflected in financial markets, with dramatic movements in stock prices and the outflow of capital from more vulnerable economies. The rapid integration through GVCs, enabled through the rapid evolution of information technology and finer degrees of specialization, have increased the exposure to external demand

and supply shocks, in a way that is far deeper than even the 2008–2009 global financial crisis, though the latter provides an instructive "benchmark" against which to examine the magnitude of the COVID-19 economic crisis that is only now unfolding.

Like the Great Depression, the global financial crisis began largely as a financial market crisis in a single country (see Figure 3.1). Accumulating defaults on mortgages and derivative products in the United States resulted in the collapse of US financial institutions causing the collapse of equity markets as the financial contagion spread. The knock-on impacts on industrial production spread across advanced economies and spilled over to emerging markets and developing countries, particularly those integrated into GVCs. The 2008 financial crisis caused a precipitous fall in GDP across four-fifths of the world and resulted in rising unemployment.

COVID-19's Economic contagion and transmission mechanisms

COVID-19's global economic impact

The engines of growth in the Western economy – the United States, Europe – are and will be deeply affected by the COVID-19 economic crisis. As the virus spreads internationally, developed countries are already taking action to limit the spread through social isolation policies, limiting work, and restricting the mobility of people. First, the crisis has simultaneously affected the largest trading nations. The epicenter of the crisis had shifted from China, the second-largest economy in late 2019, to the United States, the largest trading nation, by the end of March 2020. The top trading nations that account for 80% of world trade have contracted 70% world contagion (see Figure 3.2). Even if containment measures are limited temporally to two quarters, the propagation effects and reverberations will likely be strong, impacting developing and emerging markets that rely on advanced economy markets.

Despite being the world's second-largest economy, China's production initially plunged at the sharpest pace in three decades; it is likely to hit an upswing very quickly as the import requirements from the rest of the world land at its doorsteps. Taking advantage of the drastically lower energy prices, China can quickly ramp up its production capacity and flood the market to meet the unmet demand (trade, finance, commodity prices, and tourism), compounding the toll on developing countries.[2]

On a global scale, the economic contagion is projected to contract global GDP by 3% in 2020 (IMF, April 2020), much worse in comparison to the global financial crisis, during which the global economy contracted by 2% in 2009 (UN, 2010). Maliszewska et al. (2020) estimated economic outcomes of an "amplified global pandemic" where they assume all major countries' output contraction mimic that of China (December 2019–January 2020) but experiencing a deeper and prolonged pandemic. The result would be a 2.1% fall in global GDP in the

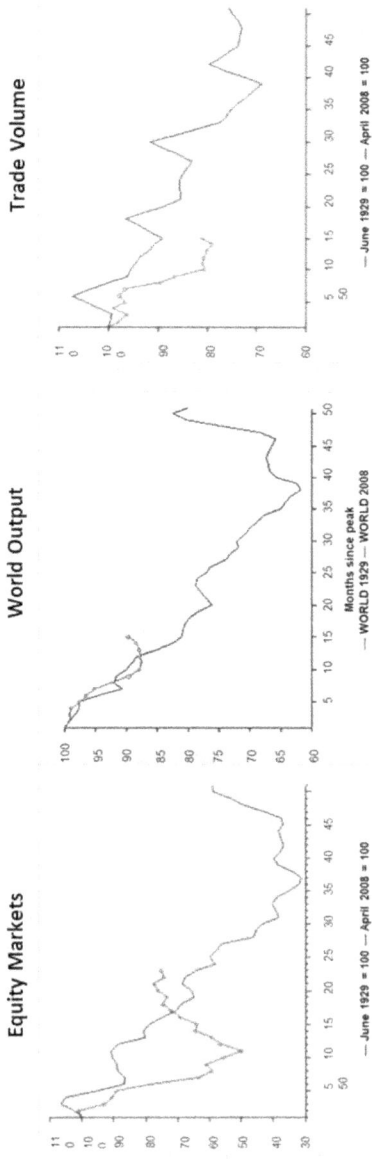

Figure 3.1 Global Impact of Financial Crisis and Great Depression on Economic Indicators.

Source: Eichengreen and Rourke (2010).

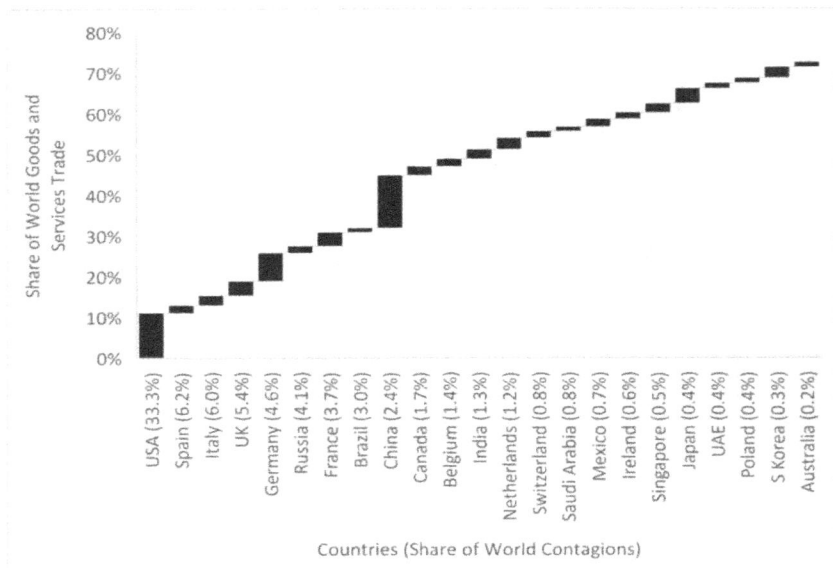

Figure 3.2 Contagion Share of Major Traders as of May 4, 2020.

Source: Author's calculations using World Bank's WDI data.

short term, with high-income countries dipping by 1.9% and developing countries by 2.5%. The IMF forecasts that if the pandemic fades in the second half of 2020 and containment efforts can be gradually unwound, with significant policy support by advanced, developing, and emerging markets, the global economy is expected to return to growth by 5.8% in 2021 (IMF, April 2020).

COVID's impact on global trade flows

The latest global level real-time estimates show a dramatic weakness in trade. The real-time estimates of world trade for exports and imports (Figure 3.3) show that, as China started reopening its economy after the lockdown, world exports initially recovered across the board. The heterogeneous effects at the sectoral level, classified by broad vessel categories, show oil and related product performance is especially strong but is not fully matched by an increase in world imports – in line with reports that crude oil is being stored at sea. Beginning mid-March, the trend reversed for less commoditized goods (those transported in containers and finished vehicles) started to dip dramatically (Figure 3.4), a consequence of companies halting production and households postponing purchases of durable goods (Table 3.1).

The 2008 financial crisis, which originated in the United States and rapidly spread through multiple channels to low- and middle-income countries,

Table 3.1 IMF Growth Forecast

Countries and regions	Projections		
	2019	*2020*	*2021*
World output	2.9	−3.0	5.8
Advanced economies	1.7	−6.1	4.5
United States	2.3	−5.9	4.7
Euro Area	1.2	−7.5	4.7
Germany	0.6	−7.0	5.2
France	1.3	−7.2	4.5
Italy	0.3	−9.1	4.8
Spain	2.0	−8.0	4.3
Japan	0.7	−5.2	3.0
United Kingdom	1.4	−6.5	4.0
Canada	1.6	−6.2	4.2
Other advanced economies	1.7	−4.6	4.5
Emerging market and developing economies	3.7	−1	6.6
Emerging and developing Asia	5.5	1.0	8.5
China	6.1	1.2	9.2
India	4.2	1.9	7.4
ASEAN-54	4.8	−0.6	7.8
European Union	1.7	−7.1	4.8
Low-income developing countries	5.1	0.4	5.6
World trade volume (goods and services)	0.9	−11	8.4
Imports			
Advanced economies	1.5	−11.5	7.5
Emerging market and developing economies	−0.8	−8.2	9.1
Exports			
Advanced economies	1.2	−12.8	7.4
Emerging market and developing economies	0.8	−9.6	11

Source: World Economic Outlook (WEO), IMF (2020).

offers a few clues of the extent of the impending COVID-19-related trade contraction. Global trade volumes fell from the end of 2008 through the first half of 2009 as a result of declining imports by developed countries, especially in the United States, which accounted for 15% of the global total (United Nations, 2010). At the height of the crisis, between July 2008 and April 2009, the value of imports of the EU, Japan, and the United States plummeted by almost 40% and triggered a worldwide collapse in international trade. The volume of imports of the three major developed economies fell by about 18% during that period, a situation which was compounded by a decline of about 24% in import prices. The developing countries experienced a rapid 25% decline in exports from 2008 to 2009 before recovering in 2010. Despite the gradual recovery during the ensuing period, the value of imports of the three largest developed economies was still about 25% below pre-crisis peaks by August 2010.

The trade never returned to its previous trend, represented by the dotted grey line (Figure 3.5). The trade elasticity (the ratio of trade growth to GDP growth)

(Real time estimates of world trade relative to 2017-19 average)

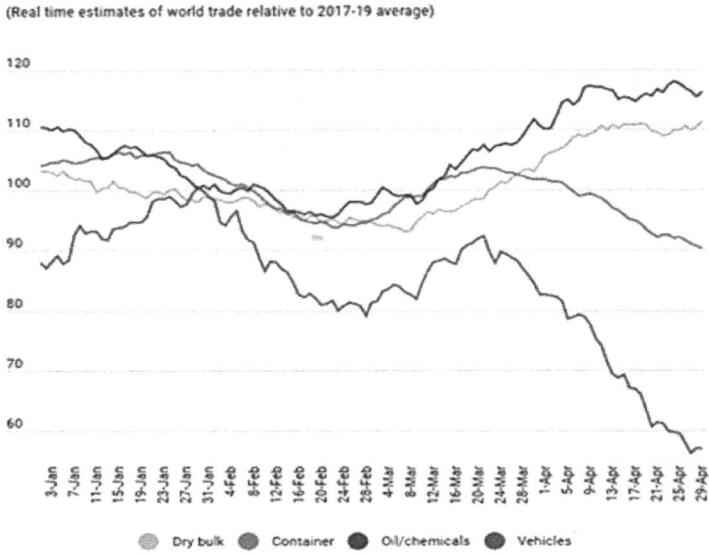

Figure 3.3 Post-COVID-19 Exports.

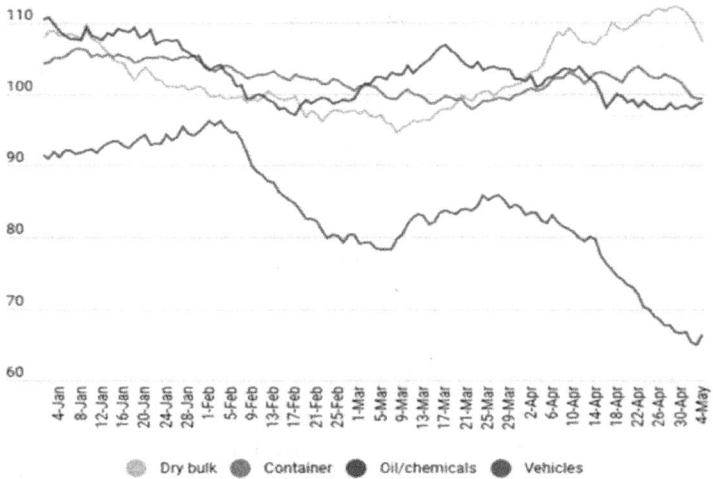

Note: 30-day moving averages. The methodology is only designed to track trade in goods.

Figure 3.4 Post-COVID-19 Imports.

Source: Cerdeiro, Komaromi, Liu and Saeed (2020); AIS data from Marine Traffic.

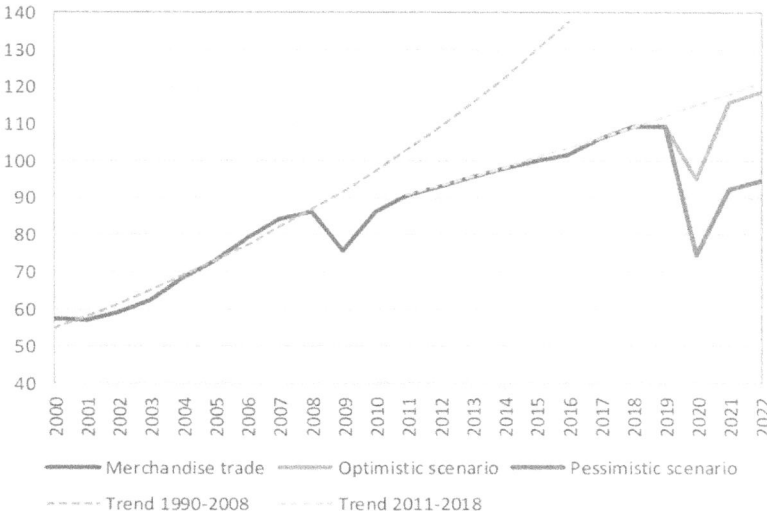

Figure 3.5 World Merchandise Trade Volume, 2000–2022 (index, 2015 = 100).

Source: UNWTO, (2020).

in the 1990s was greater than two (Bekkers et al., 2020). After the financial crisis, trade growth slowed, and trade elasticity declined, even below its long-term average. The trade slowdown was more structural change in the relationship between trade and income than merely cyclical (Constantinescu et al., 2015). First, high-income countries, which accounted for some 70% of global imports, remained weak after the financial crisis. Second, the structure of GVCs that previously propagated world trade shifted, with a higher proportion of the value of final goods being added domestically, reducing the number of links in the chain and, therefore, trade volumes.

Several different modeling efforts over the past months have yielded various scenarios for the impact of COVID-19 on aggregate demand and trade flows. IMF estimates suggest that, in the aggregate, world import demand in 2020 is expected to contract by 11%, led by the advanced economies, and exports of emerging and developing countries contracting by 9.6% (IMF, April 2020). Using Computable General Equilibrium (CGE) modeling at regional/income aggregates, WTO (2020), (Table 3.2) projections show North America's (primarily the United States) and EU imports would experience a double-digit dip in 2020, even under an optimistic scenario, declining as much as 33% and 29%, respectively, under a more pessimistic scenario.[3] The 2021 projections suggest a rapid recovery from the second half of 2020. In the aggregate, World Tourism Organization (WTO) estimates that developing country exports show a similar consistency in merchandise trade reductions for 2020, between 10% and 31%, with a double-digit

Table 3.2 Merchandise Trade Volumes and Real GDP, 2018–2021 (Annual % Change)

	Historical		*Optimistic scenario*		*Pessimistic scenario*	
	2018	*2019*	*2020*	*2021*	*2020*	*2021*
Volume of merchandise world trade	2.9	−0.1	−12.9	21.3	−31.9	24
Exports						
North America	3.8	1.0	−17.1	23.7	−40.9	19.3
South and Central America	0.1	−2.2	−12.9	18.6	−31.3	14.3
Europe	2.0-	0.1	−12.2	20.5	−32.8	22.7
Asia	3.7	0.9	−13.5	24.9	−36.2	36.1
Other regions	0.7	−2.9	−8.0	8.6	−8.0	9.3
Imports						
North America	5.2	−0.4	−14.5	27.3	−33.8	29.5
South and Central America	5.3	−2.1	−22.2	23.2	−43.8	19.5
Europe	1.5	0.5	−10.3	19.9	−28.9	24.5
Asia	4.9	10.6	−11.8	23.1	−31.5	35.1
Other regions	0.3	1.5	−10.0	13.6	−22.6	18.0

Source: WTO (2020).

recovery in 2022. The World Bank's East Asia Update, under an "amplified" global pandemic scenario, shows several countries that experience larger than global average losses of exports are in the East Asia and Pacific, including China (9%), Cambodia (7.4%), Laos (7%), Thailand (6.8%) and the Philippines (6.4%) (World Bank, 2020a,b,c), Table 3.3. In the amplified global spread of the virus, all countries see their total exports decline, but the less integrated countries in the Middle East, North Africa, and Sub-Saharan Africa are expected to be the least affected. The initial shock similarly affects all sectors, by limiting the availability of labor and capital, though labor-intensive sectors are likely to be hit harder.

Table 3.3 Real Exports Impacts of COVID-19 (Cumulative Impacts, % Deviations from the Benchmark)

Countries	*Pandemic*	*Amplified pandemic*
China	−3.73	−3.08
Cambodia	−3.89	−7.40
Laos	−3.57	−7.29
Malaysia	−2.45	−5.28
Thailand	−3.40	−6.81
Vietnam	−1.00	−2.82
Philippines	−2.94	−6.35
Indonesia	−1.38	−3.21
Sub-Saharan Africa	−1.87	−4.29
Brazil	−2.03	−4.27
India	−1.68	−3.45
Rest of South Asia	−1.99	−4.12

Source: East Asia Update, World Bank (2020a,b,c).

Economic contagion through trade

The extent and the way a country is integrated into the global economy, will determine the severity of the crisis in different countries. Developing countries are deeply entrenched with developed countries through trade. This includes the impact of the crisis on aggregate demand for both goods and services, particularly the impact through GVCs, through reduced earnings from tourism, and the impact on commodity markets. They will also be impacted due to financial market instability and the flow of remittances, which are an important source of foreign reserves and serve as a de-facto social safety net for many. A protracted downturn can also affect the direction and volume of foreign direct investment flows, which, in turn, can shape their future economic growth and structure.

The following sections discuss some of these key transmission mechanisms for COVID-19 economic contagion, including lessons learned from previous economic crises.

Transmission through increased trade costs

Trade costs impact trade in goods that rely heavily on imported inputs and the service sectors that contribute to the value-added of goods, such as call centers, product design, and after-sales service. For example, IT and business services in India are strongly tied to global manufacturing, even if these services are not all directly exported. For example, in India, business and IT are exported as part of business process outsourcing (BPO) and the domestic value added as a share of the country's total exports (18%). Sri Lanka's domestic value-added in transport as a share of total exports is equal to 12%.

COVID-19 is likely to increase trade costs than the previous crisis – some of this is already evident. Transport and other transaction costs in foreign trade include not only the cost of transportation but also the costs created by additional inspections, reduced hours of operation at ports of entry and/or border closures, as well as road closures. The ongoing lockdowns and social distancing–prompted restrictions on movement to slow the spread of the disease mean that transport and travel were directly affected in ways they were not during the global financial crisis. The Ebola outbreak in 2014 is estimated to have increased trade costs in affected countries by 10% (Evans et al., 2014). Since COVID-19 is affecting more countries and the containment measures are more severe and widespread due to the efforts to contain the virus, Bekkers et al. (2020) estimated that, in the case of an amplified shock due to COVID-19, it would increase international trade costs of imports and exports, for most countries, by about 25%.

Formal estimates are dwarfed by real-time anecdotal evidence. First, high-frequency shipping data for the first part of April showed major reductions in capacity on the main sea trade lines, signaling reductions in container throughput (World Bank, 2020a,b,c). The reduction in capacity is more significant for Europe-Asia routes than trans-Pacific routes, amounting to 33% and 13% reductions, respectively. The sharp decline in aviation connectivity represents substantial reductions in airborne shipping capacity, as well. Half of all air cargo travels as "belly cargo" in passenger planes also impacted the worldwide travel restrictions – the decline in global passenger flights, which began in February, accelerated in March and April, dropping 59.2% in the week of April 8, 2020. Seabury/Accenture reported global air cargo capacity dropped 35% (Seabury, 2020).

The unprecedented limited belly capacity in passenger planes has led to a dramatic reduction in air freight space availability (Figure 3.6), fueling a very lopsided competition of merchants trying to ship their product versus the urgently needed orders of large quantities of personal protective equipment (PPE), which require fulfillment by air. This has caused airfreight prices to rise dramatically, especially the trans-Pacific trade lane. China to North America spot airfreight pricing exceeded US$10 per kilogram by May, and full freighters are selling above US$1 mil per flight. Air shipments from London to New York that may have previously had an airfreight cost of US$3,500 increased ten-fold by the end of April (Relocation Plus, n.d.). The temporary rise in demand for PPE has kept several key cargo fleets afloat despite the costs. However, the limited capacity is likely to linger as countries clamor to compete for space, putting further pressure on prices. Since the demand for PPE will remain strong for the foreseeable future, the elevated prices for airfreight are not expected to drop until COVID-19 has been contained.

With higher trade costs, the price per unit of cargo increases – substantially in the case of GVC-related trade where parts and components may be sourced from multiple countries, as well as for low-value, bulky items. The rising trade costs represent a productivity loss since additional resources are needed to bring goods to consumers instead of being available for investment or other productivity-enhancing measures. In some cases, exports of medical supplies and food have been banned, while shortages of parts and components have interrupted production in industries characterized by complex value chains.

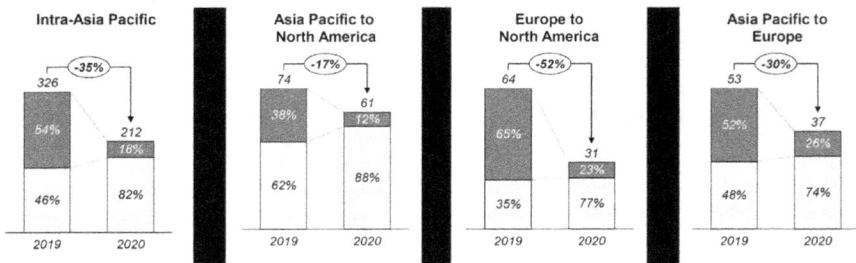

Figure 3.6 Inter-Regional Cargo Capacity Comparison, 2019 vs. 2020.

Source: (Seabury, 2020). Note: Gray = Freight, Blue = Passenger.

Transmission through GVCs

The world is as interconnected as never before through intricate production and services linkages within GVCs. The hardest hit initially was China and South Korea – both critical to the flow of parts and components and assembly. The second wave of contagion hit the EU, United States, and Japan – all central to both the supply and demand for GVC-related products and services. The most affected countries account for about 80% of global trade and include all dominant and essential nodes of the global economic system (see Figure 3.7). The advanced countries at the core of the network, simultaneously locked down, are essential to the world trading system and developing and emerging markets. Some developing countries such as Bangladesh and Sri Lanka are directly connected to consumption nodes in the United States and United Kingdom through the apparel sector, with backward linkages to East Asia, where textiles may be sourced. Others, such as Thailand's automotive sector, are connected via central nodes in China and Japan, from which advanced components are sourced and final goods are exported. Still other developing countries, for example, in Sub-Saharan Africa, supply raw materials to others along the value chain, such as bauxite and tantalum – so-called forward linkages.

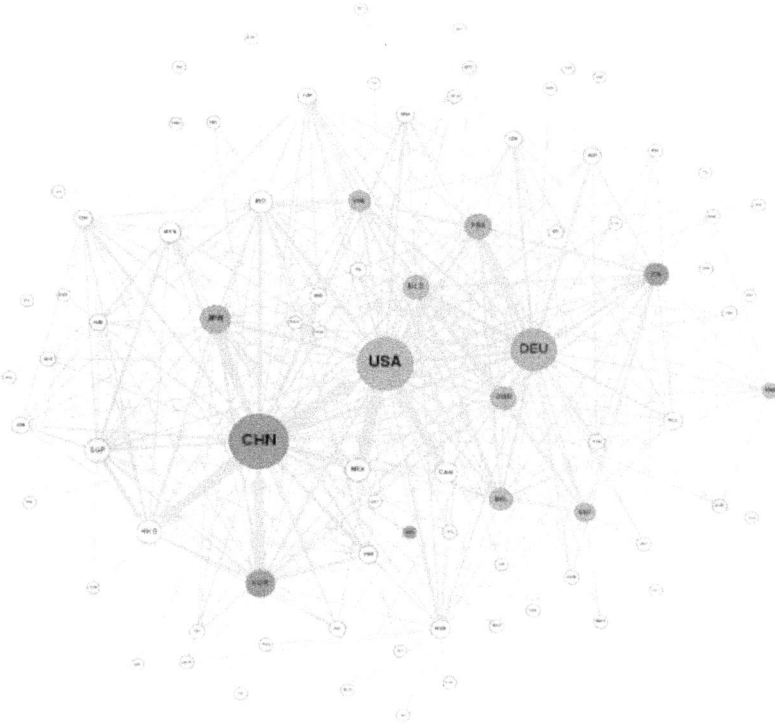

Figure 3.7 Global Network of Intermediate Trade, 2018.

HIGH GVC FORWARD LINKAGES INCREASE EXPOSURE TO DEMAND SHOCKS

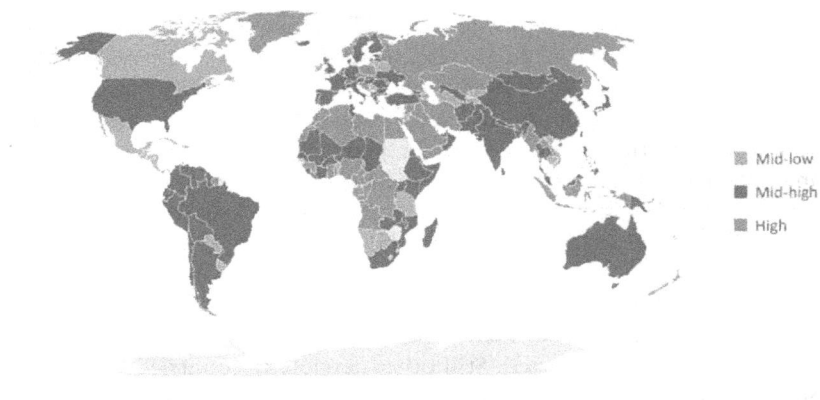

Figure 3.8 GVC Forward Linkages.

Source: World Development Report (2020)

Beyond the increased transport costs, developing and emerging markets that are linked through global supply chains are affected by the crisis in two principal ways. First is the ***demand shock***, through a precipitous collapse of consumption of so-called "postponables," i.e. purchases that can be delayed – as seen in the trade collapse of 2009, the wait-and-see demand shock impacted durable goods more than non-durable goods. Reductions in demand lead to a "bullwhip" effect, whereby a collapse in demand for final goods leads each producer/supplier along the chain to discharge their inventories before re-ordering. Consequently, the demand shock gets amplified for suppliers further up the supply chain, including both intermediate goods producers and raw material suppliers (Zavacka, 2012).

These demand shocks have, due to lockdowns and reduced transport capacity, been coupled with ***supply-side shocks***. The WDR 2020 finds that developing countries that specialize in manufacturing tend to integrate predominantly via backward linkages in the global economy, i.e. they import large amounts of inputs from abroad that they use to produce their exports (Figure 3.8). Backward linkages make a country susceptible to supply shocks since vital sources of inputs may be shut down or countries start imposing export restrictions. Under the current crisis, firms of key intermediate suppliers across the globe shuttered their workplaces, reducing the production of goods, including those for which demand remains. Like the case of a demand-side shock, such supply shocks have reverberated down supply chains and will be particularly acute

HIGH GVC BACKWARD LINKAGES MEAN THAT COUNTRIES ALSO NEED TO WORRY ABOUT SUPPLY SHOCKS

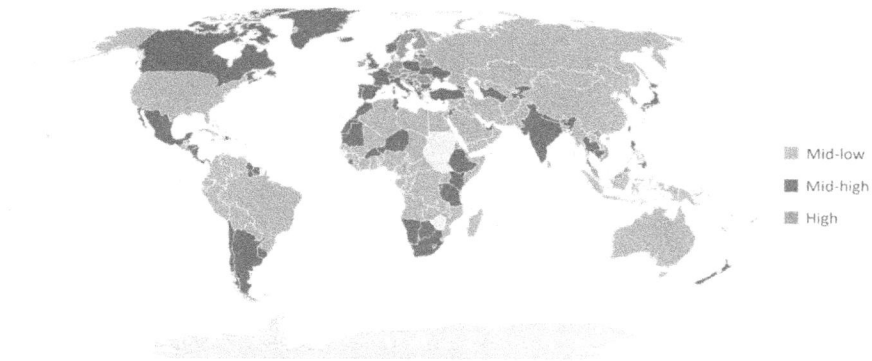

Mid-low

Mid-high

High

Figure 3.9 GVC Backward Linkages.

Source: World Development Report (2020).

in sectors that rely on just-in-time inventories. Therefore, supply-chain contagion will amplify the direct supply shocks as manufacturing sectors, even in less-affected nations, find it harder and/or more expensive to acquire the necessary imported industrial inputs from the hard-hit nations and subsequently from each other (Figure 3.9).

While value chain disruptions due to COVID-19 were initially confined to China – which sits at the nexus of many GVCs, as either (or both) supplier or final producer – once the pandemic becomes more widespread, trade can be expected to fall more steeply in sectors characterized by complex value chain linkages, particularly in electronics, pharmaceutical, and automotive products. Even localized disruptions such as hurricanes, tsunamis, and other crises can also affect complex value chains, as demonstrated by the March 2011 tsunami that forced Japanese corporations in the United States to halt production as they were unable to obtain parts and components from their suppliers in Japan.

Transmission through foreign direct investment

Changes in trade flows can, for some countries, become more permanent, transforming from an episodic downturn to a more generalized reduction in capacity and/or structural shifts, both through insolvencies and reductions in foreign investment to other countries that are better positioned to rebound from the crisis. COVID-19 has created uncertainty in global capital flows, with a massive outflow of capital from developing countries to safer havens. COVID-19 also has implications on how global investment flows will behave as emergency clears. Foreign investment has historically been a barometer of developing countries' health and their ability to grow and integrate with the global economy. While the immediate crisis has frozen new investments, a specter looms on the horizon once the health emergency subsides, with some multinationals seeking to re-shore operations that can be automated or shifting investments to other countries to lower their future risk portfolio. This may have long-lasting effects on developing countries that will compete for a shrinking volume of foreign investment.

In the light of COVID-19, the United Nations Conference on Trade and Development (UNCTAD) recently revised its forecasts on global FDI flows from a conservative 5 to 15% drop to a decisive 30 to 40% decline during 2020–2021. During the financial crisis of 2007–2008 and its immediate aftermath, FDI flows fell by 37% in 2009, down to US$1.1 trillion. Today, at the onset of the pandemic, the crisis has already wiped off some US$500 billion in foreign investment, and worse, it is more likely to emerge as earnings are downgraded (United Nations Conference on Trade and Development – UNCTAD, 2020).

Earnings guidance by multinational enterprises (MNEs) in UNCTAD's top 100, which rely on their foreign direct investments for an average of 50% of reinvested earnings, confirms the rapid deterioration of FDI outflow prospects. Some 61% of the MNEs have issued new statements since the first week of March. In addition to earlier concerns of supply disruptions from China, 57% have warned of the global demand shock's impact on sales, showing that COVID-19 is causing problems beyond supply chain disruptions. Besides, the top 5,000 MNEs, which account for a significant share of global FDI, have now seen downward revisions of 30% on average for 2020 earnings estimates – these sentiments were yet to capture the sudden spike in COVID-19 cases in the United States, which is likely to depress earnings further. The most affected sectors are energy and primary metals industries, with an expected 200+ percent decline in earnings (see the section below on the impact of commodity markets), airlines (116% decline), and the automotive industry, which faces both demand- and supply-side shocks (47% decline).

The negative impact is likely to reverberate across upstream and downstream supply chain investments across Asia, Central and Southern Europe, and South America, with more enduring effects on production networks. Even without further downward revisions, those losses are potentially more dramatic than at any time in modern history. The implications will range from delays in investments with long gestation periods to projects that are downsized or shelved indefinitely, including the abandonment of mergers and acquisitions – all of which may accelerate trends already in motion pre-COVID-19 to shift GVC-related operations back home to reduce supply chain risks. This also has the potential to weaken the future competitiveness of developing countries that may find it more difficult to bring in private capital to finance much-needed energy infrastructure projects.

Tourism Receipts and as share of total exports (2018)

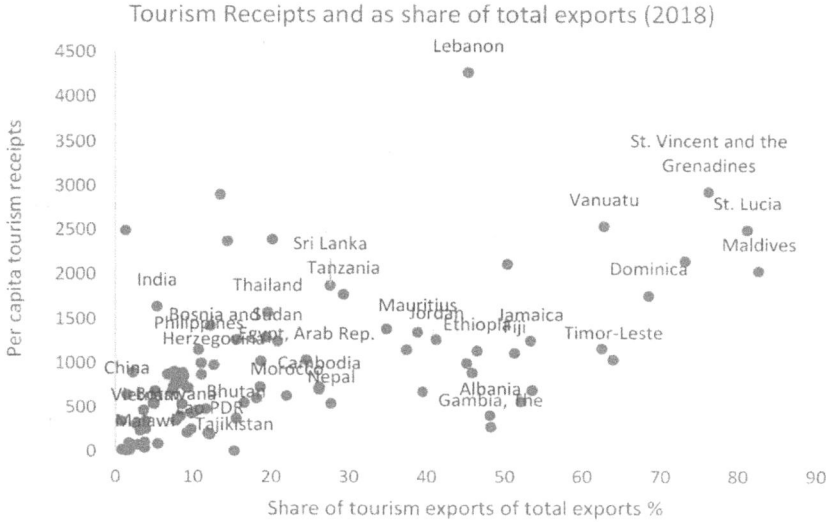

Figure 3.10 Tourism Receipts as a Share of Exports.

Source: World Bank's WDI data.

Transmission through the tourism sector

Economic contagion to developing and emerging markets will also be transmitted through trade in services. Some services may benefit from the crisis – this is true of information technology services, demand for which has boomed as companies try to enable employees to work from home and socialize remotely. However, with the imposition of transport and travel restrictions and the closure of many retail and hospitality establishments, the services trade will take its own toll especially on countries tourism receipts are larger share of exports (see Figure 3.10). Services are not included in the WTO's merchandise trade forecast, but most trade in goods would be impossible without them (e.g. transport). Unlike goods, there are no inventories of services to be drawn down today and restocked at a later stage. As a result, declines in services trade during the pandemic may be lost forever. Services are also interconnected, with air transport enabling an ecosystem of other cultural, sporting, and recreational activities.

Tourism receipts are essential for all economies but constitute a critical share of total exports (and foreign exchange earnings) for developing and emerging market economies and, in particular, for small-island economies. For Maldives, Jamaica, and St. Lucia, for example, tourism constitutes over two-thirds of exports and GDP and around 40% of government revenues.

Tourism supports a multitude of direct and indirect livelihoods than just direct tourism receipts and indirect and induced impacts through capital spending, government spending, and supply-chain activities, such as purchases of domestic and imported goods and services. Using a broadened definition to accommodate both indirect and induced impacts, satellite accounts and input-output tables show the overall impact on the economy tourism is important even for large countries and those that surround them (and are often part of multi-country itineraries) – for example, tourism accounts for over 9% of India's GDP and generate significant spillovers to Nepal, Bhutan, and Sri Lanka.

As of May 5, 2020, 96% of worldwide destinations introduced travel restrictions in response to the pandemic (see Figure 3.11) (UNWTO, 2020). Of these, 90 destinations completely or partially closed their borders and 44 destinations have introduced travel bans for passengers coming from selected destinations that have been affected by COVID-19, and 56 destinations suspended all or partially international flights into the destination (see Figure 3.11). International tourism was down by 22% in Q1 and is expected to decline by 60 to 80%, compared with 2019 – an US$80 billion decline in exports. On 24 March, UNWTO estimated international tourist arrivals would decline by 20% to 30% in 2020, back to the levels of 5 to 7 years ago. This would translate into a loss of US$250 to US$400 billion in international tourism receipts – almost a third of the US$1.5 trillion generated globally.

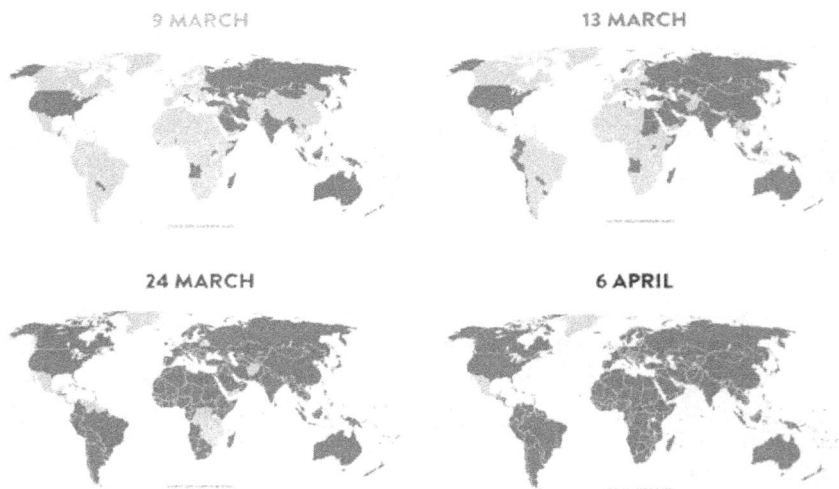

Figure 3.11 Timeline of Pandemic's Effects of Global Tourism.

Source: UNWTO (2020).

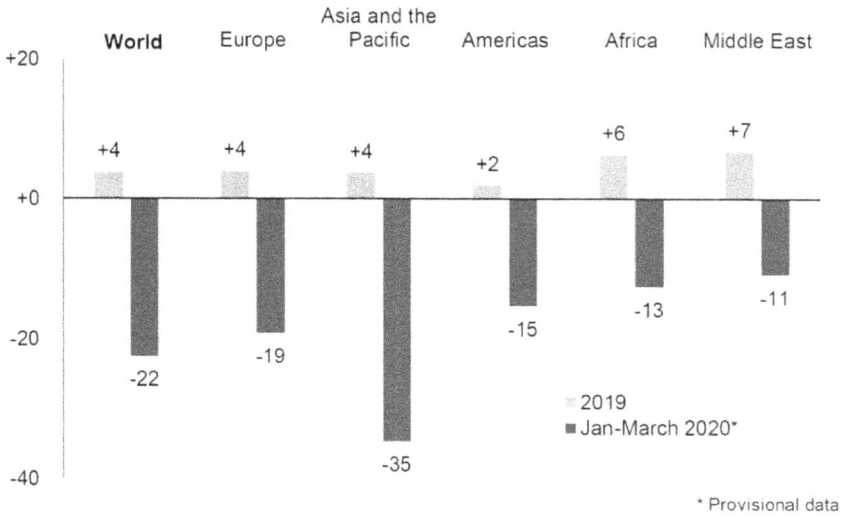

Figure 3.12 International Tourist Arrivals, 2019 and Q1 2020 (% Change).

Source: UNWTO (2020).

Covid-19 has dramatically affected tourism arrivals (See Figure 3.12). As of May, tourism around most parts of the world – especially in Europe, Asia, and Sub-Saharan Africa – is at a virtual freeze, with some stranded tourists gradually being allowed back into their origin countries. As the uncertainty of the pandemic continues to evolve, the UN World Tourism Organization (UNWTO) estimates project a 58 to 78% decline in tourism arrivals for 2020. UNWTO estimates forecast that the Asia and Pacific region will suffer the highest decline in relative and absolute terms (a loss of 33 million arrivals); the impact in Europe, though lower in percentage, is quite high in volume (22 million arrivals). The decline in tourism revenues will affect most Cambodia, Lao PDR, Malaysia, Pacific Islands, the Philippines, and Thailand – in each, tourism revenues constitute more than 10% of GDP. Fiji, Kiribati, Palau, Samoa, and Vanuatu are the most exposed to tourism. COVID-19 will hurt commodity and tourism revenues and disrupt imports of raw materials and inflows of workers for infrastructure projects in many small island economies.

UNWTO's simulation extends the likely scenario under three conditions: (1) gradual opening of international borders and easing of travel restrictions, with 58% of destinations open in early July, (2) 70% opening in early September, and (3) 78% of destinations delaying to early December. Under the latter, the result

A. Commodity price indices, monthly

Index, 100 = 2010

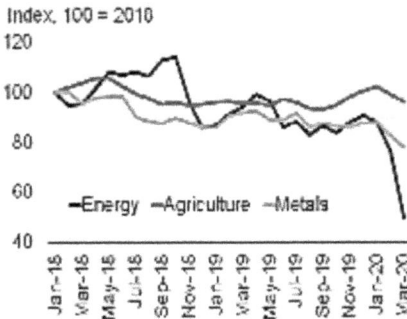

—Energy —Agriculture —Metals

B. Commodity price changes since January 20th

Percent

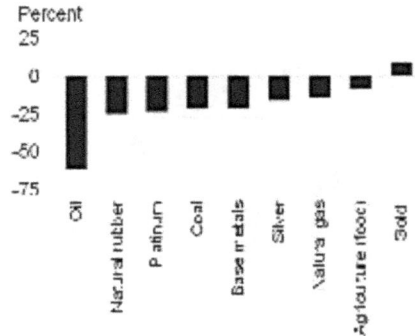

Figure 3.13 Commodity Price Indices.

Source: World Bank Commodity Market Outlook (2020).

would be a loss of 850 million to 1.1 billion international tourists, totaling a loss of US$910 billion to US$1.2 trillion in export revenues and 100 to 120 million direct tourism jobs globally. A rebound is expected, however, in 2021, with domestic demand within countries expected to recover faster than international demand and leisure travel faster than business travel, particularly for visiting friends and relatives (Figure 3.13).

Transmission through commodity markets

Commodity markets have also been shaken by the ongoing crisis, which will have both immediate and ongoing impacts on commodity prices and, in turn, will have spillover effects on other traded sectors, incomes, and government revenues. Commodity markets have been and will be largely driven by demand-side factors, though supply-side disruptions may have spillover impacts on prices, such as through the same transport-related costs that are expected to impact GVCs, particularly for low unit value agricultural commodities.

The impact of lockdowns and other mitigation measures have caused virtually all commodity prices to decline sharply. Reduced transport and manufacturing have brought down energy prices dramatically as the pandemic spread – crude oil prices dropped 50% between January and March 2020 – and are expected to continue to decline in the face of reduced economic activity. Metals and other industrial minerals are following suit. On the other hand, most agricultural commodity prices have been more stable, as they are less sensitive to economic activity and stocks of staple crops are at an all-time high. Nevertheless, in the short run, disruptions to agricultural supply chains – and increased transport

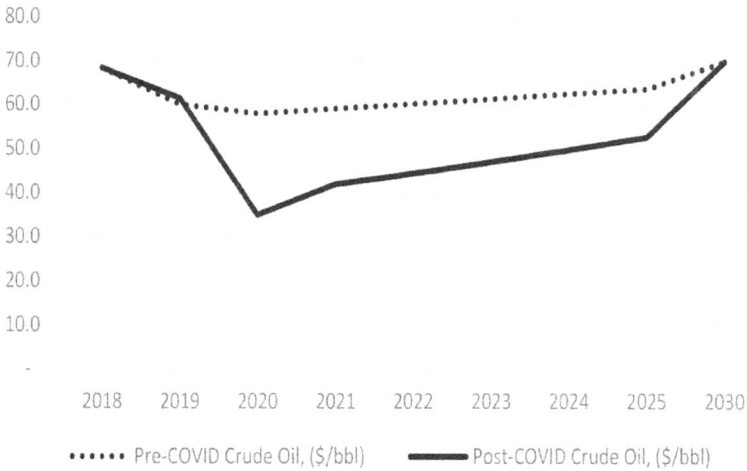

Figure 3.14 Crude Oil Price Forecast.

Source: World Bank Commodity Market Outlook (2020).

costs – could imperil food security and rural livelihoods in developing countries that could, in turn, foment further instability in regions that are already security hotspots (Figure 3.14). The path to price recovery will likely vary significantly across commodities, with varying impacts on trade and economic growth outcomes in countries dependent on either their import or export – far greater shifts than other economic recessions or disruptions and longer-term impacts on trade and incomes.

The impact of COVID-19 has already taken a significant toll on energy prices, particularly crude oil. While spot prices dropped rapidly from January, US futures took an unprecedented fall in April, dropping for the first time below zero as overproduction and the sudden drop in demand together took their toll, as producers were forced to pay to dispose of excess production. Despite commitments by OPEC, the United States, Canada, and other oil-producing countries, it is expected that oil prices will be exceptionally slow to recover, with forecasted prices remaining below pre-COVID price trends through 2025 and beyond, following a similar but more dramatic path than experienced after previous price collapses, such as the 1997 and 2008/2009 financial crises, the 1986 OPEC price collapse, and the more recent 2016 collapse. History strongly suggests that it is not likely that OPEC+ and other large oil-producing countries will be able to shore up prices enough to offset the downward pressure from reduced global demand (Figure 3.15).

While the collapse in oil prices will benefit many oil-importing developing countries, offsetting, at least partially, the decline in real incomes, exporting

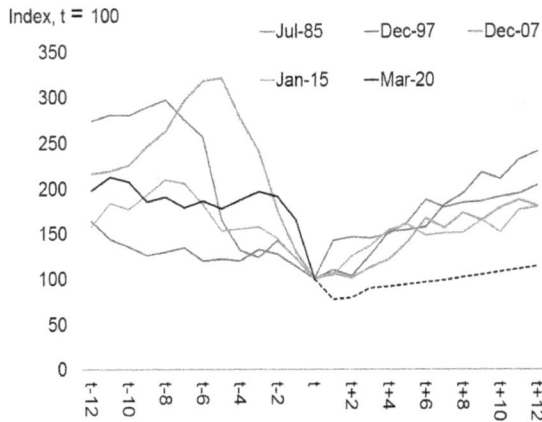

Figure 3.15 Oil Price Recovery Trends.

Source: World Bank Commodity Market Outlook (2020).

developing countries – some already facing instability before the crisis (e.g. Venezuela, Nigeria, and Angola) – will find their primary source of foreign reserves severely constrained and reducing government revenues desperately needed to address the immediate crisis and stimulate recovery.

The price fluctuations on non-energy minerals will vary considerably. While precious metals will benefit from investors' flight to safe-haven assets, industrial metals, except for iron ore, are already under pressure from decreased demand, with expected drops in prices in 2020 and continued decline through 2025. Nickel and zinc are forecast to fall 22% in 2020 (Figure 3.16) and tin, copper, and lead will fall between 13% and 17%. A number of developing countries across South and Southeast Asia, Sub-Saharan Africa, and Latin America are significant producers and will be negatively impacted, causing a similar fall in foreign reserves of domestic revenue mobilization. Like crude oil, prices of some, such as copper and nickel are not expected to recover their pre-COVID levels until after 2025.

Selected developing country commodity exporters

Bauxite/aluminum – Guinea, Brazil, India, Indonesia
    Lead – Peru, India, Bolivia
    Nickel – Indonesia, Philippines
    Tin – Indonesia, Myanmar, Peru
    Zinc – Peru, India, Bolivia

While only a relatively small number of developing countries are significant producers of metal and mineral commodities, virtually all rely heavily on agriculture

Industrial Metals

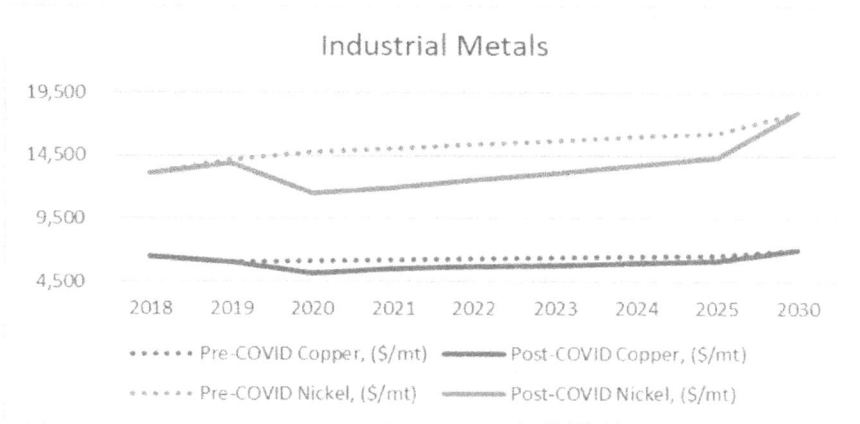

19,500

14,500

9,500

4,500

2018   2019   2020   2021   2022   2023   2024   2025   2030

• • • • • • Pre-COVID Copper, ($/mt)   ▬▬▬ Post-COVID Copper, ($/mt)

• • • • • • Pre-COVID Nickel, ($/mt)   ▬▬▬ Post-COVID Nickel, ($/mt)

Figure 3.16 Industrial Metal Prices, Pre- and Post-COVID.

Source: World Bank Commodity Market Outlook (2020).

to support livelihoods. As the crisis subsides, most commodity prices will likely stabilize as the demand-shock subsides and food stockpiles are diminished, and a reduction in input prices, such as fertilizers and energy, which were already in decline pre-COVID. Cash crops such as cocoa, coffee, and tea are expected to rebound relatively quickly, with positive growth returning in 2021. Downstream sectors such as palm and groundnut oil will also remain strong, with positive growth prevailing even in 2020. The greatest risk to the food sector is likely to be transmitted through supply chain disruptions that slow the movement

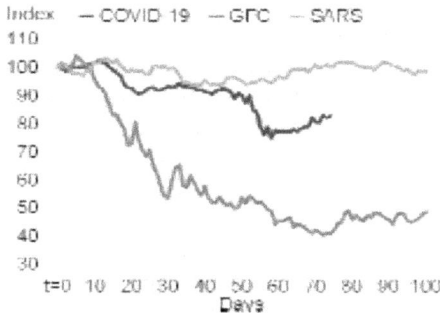

Index   — COVID-19   — GFC   — SARS

110
100
90
80
70
60
50
40
30

t=0 10 20 30 40 50 60 70 80 90 100
Days

Figure 3.17 Copper Price Trends in Crisis.

Source: World Bank Commodity Market Outlook (2020).

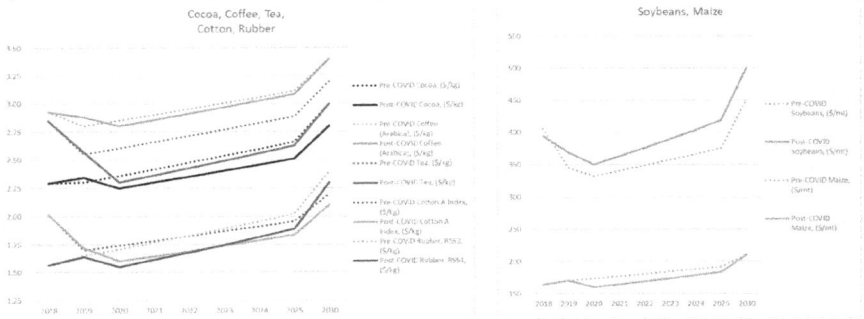

Figure 3.18 Agricultural Commodity Price Forecast, Pre- and Post-COVID.

Source: World Bank Commodity Market Outlook (2020).

of agricultural commodities within and between countries. For example, both Argentina and Brazil faced shutdowns and blockades of key transport infrastructure within and at the ports. Future outbreaks have the potential to exacerbate these logistical challenges (Figure 3.17) and (Figure 3.18).

Concluding remarks and a few policy options

Under most conservative estimates, i.e. the best-case scenario, the advanced countries are unlikely to return to pre-COVID-19 aggregate demand before the fourth quarter of 2021. Even when the crisis bottoms out, widespread bankruptcies increased unemployment and under-employment, and a depressed investment climate across much of Sri Lanka's major trading partners would result in smaller merchandise and service markets in the short-term, requiring new and innovative approaches and business models to survive under the "New Normal."

Under the still reverberating COVID-19 crisis, export-oriented growth will likely be slow to come for Sri Lanka's economic recovery in the short-run but remains the most potent strategy for the long-term recovery and growth. The response to the crisis should not be a tradeoff between short-term expediency and long-term resiliency. In the short-run, potential options that incentivize domestic industries (through efficient industrial policy that promotes exports) may be undertaken with clearly defined objectives and criteria that generate efficiency and minimize welfare costs. Amid the downturn, rapid digitization and the servicification of the manufacturing and agricultural sectors present a window of opportunity. To harness such opportunities, national **trade policy strategies would need to be centered around encouraging new technology diffusion and enhancing human capital**. Openness to goods and services and ideas remains the conduit for access to technologies and allows countries to specialize in what they do best. Encouraging science, technology, and innovation (**STI**) **policies** through grants, credit, and tax breaks should be a cornerstone of any trade or industrial policy strategy. Trade policy may still not be the only instrument in addressing market failures when tax policy, training, and marketing are less distortionary options to choose from. Moreover, reducing constricting regulations and red-tape, inefficiencies and rent-seeking at Customs, together with soft and hard trade-related infrastructure, remains a significant part of transactions costs that affect SMEs, in particular, and should be part of a comprehensive approach to recovery and resilience.

In this context, medium- to long-term recovery needs to be centered on a pragmatic outward strategy. Sri Lanka should not miss out on forging a well thought-out FTA strategy both with larger neighbors and extended engagement with ASEAN members. Despite the COVID-19 setback, these countries remain poised to grow into the consumer markets of the future. This does not have to compromise on the existing model but complement it by reaping the efficiencies and market access, which can also stimulate FDI to further upgrade and diversify Sri Lanka's exports. The opportunity costs of complacency and inaction are likely to be substantial, especially when there is compelling evidence that transforming its long desired quest to become a maritime, logistics, and trade hub is likely to be boosted with well-designed preferential goods and services agreements with larger and fast-growing neighbors.

As far as future GVCs are concerned, some reshoring can be expected to ensure supply chain resiliency and the tendency to **regionalize GVCs closer to final demand**, as observed from the global automotive value chain. That would put further pressure on those that are still outside or on the fringes of GVCs such as Sri Lanka. The options for exports, therefore, depend on offering a distinct niche product – expanding high-end branded apparel, for example through existing relationships, leveraging unique agriculture segments to market differentiated products and quality features (such as in tea, spices, and other selected agricultural commodities), as well as services, such knowledge-process outsourcing or hub-based logistics and other services. The latter can serve new GVCs that will emerge in Asia. Differentiation takes time, but preparation can begin now. In the shorter run, global demand for PPE is expected to remain high, offering new market opportunities for those that can meet the enhanced quality control, testing, and standards to meet developed country standards.

On the **supply side,** even as some aspects of GVCs may be permanently dislocated, supply-chain risks will remain for Sri Lanka in the short term. The crisis has put into the stark light of the day the risks associated with the over-reliance on one region or country that can compromise operations. To mitigate such supply chain risks, there are three parallel initiatives that are not mutually exclusive. First, Sri Lankan producers should identify opportunities to diversify their supply base to enable rapid shifts, as needed, to address future shocks – including the likelihood of near-future COVID-19 related lockdowns.

Second, as higher-end brands and retailers in the United States and EU are likely to demand less frequent changes in styles, producers may identify opportunities to increase supply inventories. Third, as a medium- to longer-term strategy, Sri Lanka may identify opportunities to onshore selected suppliers through FDI to promote greater vertical supply chain capacity.

To emerge from the crisis, hurried **investment promotion** is unlikely to materialize results in the types of investment that will serve Sri Lanka's long-term economic development objectives. The effective handling of the COVID-19 by the government and the recovery itself would be seen favorably by the depleted pool of prospective investors. In the interim, prioritizing remaining regulatory reforms, such as streamlining investment entry and strengthening legal protections, among others, would be key. On the "soft" side, this includes streamlining and reducing the cost of market entry and reassessing incentives and tax policy. In terms of hard infrastructure, investment-ready facilities are required, including new state-of-the-art zones, industrial estates, and business parks including bio-technology parks exploring public private instruments and investment. These hard infrastructure investments will require significant investments in Sri Lanka's ability to structure public-private partnerships.

Sri Lanka also needs to look beyond its current offerings to invest in **public works and basic infrastructure,** capital investments, and measures that will serve them for the longer term and mitigate the risks associated with trade-related transmission mechanisms of future economic crises. Capital investment projects have the highest multiplier in terms of economic stimulus (versus tax cuts and/or other types of spending), creating jobs rapidly.

The Pandemic is an opportunity to rethink tourism In addition, digital technologies can be used to increase security and boost travelers' confidence. Setting up digitalization among companies and the tourism workforce, upskilling the sector to become more resilient likely to pay-off as the pandemic subsides.

Similarly, investments in other **backbone infrastructure** and accompanying policies can position Sri Lanka for the future of work and the digital age. As working from home becomes more accepted, there will be a higher demand for internet bandwidth, but also greater concerns around cybersecurity, which ultimately could push the government to boost the speed and resilience of digital infrastructure. This will need to be coupled with labor market reforms that formalize flexible work. Furthermore, platforms for contactless services will increase demand – from mobile money to e-government services to e-commerce. The latter can be a key mechanism to link smaller producers to markets, both at home and abroad. Building on the expansion of digital services such as telemedicine, mobile banking, and digital business platforms using Artificial Intelligence can produce sustained development at lower costs and high efficiency. This is also an opportunity for governments to invest in digitization and automation of government services to increase public sector efficiencies and ease the burden on private sector actors.

Notes

1. I wish to extend a special thanks to T. J. Minhas and Sheri Pitigala for review and comments.
2. A 9% contraction in China's GDP: Q1 compared the previous year and a 6% drop in US GDP in 2020: Q2. The latter is far worse than the −2.2% growth recorded in 2008: Q4. This reflects the fact that Europe and Japan were likely already heading into recession given their weak fourth-quarter performance, while the United States entered the crisis with a weakened economy. These large economies account for over 55% of world GDP and trade, and are therefore set to dramatically affect the rest of the world through various transmission mechanisms (trade, finance, commodity prices, and tourism), compounding the toll on developing countries.
3. A relatively optimistic scenario is characterized as a sharp drop in trade followed by a (V-shaped) recovery starting in the second half of 2020, and a more pessimistic scenario with a steeper initial decline and a more prolonged and incomplete (L-shaped) recovery.

References

Bekkers et al., 2020. *Trade and COVID-19: The WTO's 2020 and 2021 Trade Forecast*, EU: VOX, CEPR Policy Portal. https://voxeu.org/article/trade-and-covid-19-wto-s-2020-and-2021-trade-forecastLondon:VoxEU.org.

Constantinescu et al., 2015. The Global Trade Slowdown: Cyclical or Structural. *IMF Working Paper Series*, p. 12.

Eichengreen, B. & Rourke, K., 2010. *A Tail of Two Depressions.*

Evans, et al., 2014. *The Economic Impact of the 2014 Ebola Epidemic: Short and Medium Term Estimates for West Africa. World Bank*, (3) pp. 23–25.

IMF, April 2020. *The Great Lockdown, World Economic Outlook.* Washington, DC: s.n.

Johns Hopkins University & Medicine, 2020. International Monetary Fund. *Coronavirus Resource Center.* [Online] Available at: https://coronavirus.jhu.edu/ [Accessed 9 May 2020].

Maliszewska et al., 2020. *Potential Impact of Covid-19 on GDP and Trade.* World Bank Working Paper Series, N0: 9211 ed. Washington DC: World Bank.

Relocation Plus, n.d. *Relocation Plus.* [Online] Available at: https://www.topics.plusrelocation.com/post/102g5wa/airfreight-hitting-historic-cost-levels [Accessed 6 May 2020].

Seabury, 2020. *Global Capacity Update.* [Online] [Accessed 5 May 2020]. https://www.accenture.com/us-en/insights/travel/coronavirus-air-cargo-capacity

United Nations. 2010. *UN: World Economic Situation and Prospects 2009.* New York: UN.

UNCTAD, 2020. *Global Investment Trends Monitor.* [Online] Available at: https://unctad.org/en/PublicationsLibrary/diaeiainf2020d3_en.pdf

UNWTO, 2020. *World Tourism Barometer.* [Online] Available at: https://www.unwto.org/news/covid-19-international-tourist-numbers-could-fall-60-80-in-2020

World Bank, 2020a. *COVID-19 Trade Watch*, s.l.: World Bank. New York: Washington DC.

World Bank, 2020b. *East Asia Update.* s.l.: s.n.

World Bank, 2020c. *World Bank Indicators.* s.l.:s.n.

World Bank Group. 2020. *Commodity Markets Outlook—Persistence of Commodity Shocks, October.* World Bank, Washington, DC.

World Development Report (WDR). 2020. *Trading for Development in the Age of Global Value Chains.* World Bank: Washington, DC.

World Health Organization, 2020. *Q&A: Similarities and Differences – COVID-19 and Influenza.* [Online] Available at: https://www.who.int/emergencies/diseases/novel-coronavirus-2019/question-and-answers-hub/q-a-detail/q-a-similarities-and-differences-covid-19-and-influenza

Zavacka, V., 2012. The bullwhip effect and the great trade collapse. *European Bank for Reconstruction and Development Working Paper 148.*

4 Multilateralism and global security post-COVID-19

Thomas Wuchte and Sophie Drake

Introduction

Renewal and resurgence of multilateralism;
  A call to re-engage and to strengthen collaboration.[1]

COVID-19: A Turning Point. The COVID-19 pandemic poses an opportunity for the renewal and resurgence of global multilateral security structures, the re-engagement of leading powers, and strengthened international collaboration.

COVID-19 is a turning point. Just as the world came together in a renewed commitment to root out terrorist forces in the wake of September 11, 2001, in 2020, world powers have mobilized to combat a deadly pandemic. The mandated pause in business as usual has given time to reflect and plan (something that was not possible given the feeling of urgency following 9/11) and to determine the way forward. If the world can mobilize to such a degree in the face of a potentially cataclysmic health event, then surely the same is possible when dealing with the far more extreme crises that are to come. Non-traditional security threats, such as health crises, global poverty, and climate change, are security threats of the future. This chapter is a call to shift our understanding of security, and our framework for action, so that multilateral security organizations might view these threats with similar urgency and renewed strength. These, too, are global emergencies.

Merging old priorities with the new normal

The greatest security challenges to humankind are not always traditional warfare, or terrorism (though of course these remain significant considerations and will only be exacerbated by COVID-19[2]), but health crises, rising poverty, and climate change. These are not only threat multipliers, exacerbating existing inequalities and unrest, but they bring with them a vast range of unprecedented security issues for which our multilateral organizations are either unprepared or not placing at the forefront of their agenda. Multilateral institutions must therefore be repurposed, reprioritizing their security focus toward the imminent but harder to measure threats of the future. Multilateral organizations such as NATO and the Organization for Security and Co-operation in Europe (OSCE) ought to reconsider their spending

DOI: 10.4324/9781003197416-4

priorities, which remain focused on traditional "hard" security issues such as military preparedness and nonproliferation, arms control, disarmament, and counterterrorism. Threats such as these, while significant, can no longer be first among our multilateral security priorities. They must now give way to the unmitigable threats (if attitudes are not changed and actions not taken) of a changing climate and extreme weather, global health emergencies, and rampant poverty.

The world has needed a cohesive global response to the COVID-19 pandemic. However, multilateral institutions were not ready for this kind of non-traditional security nexus. Typically, health and climate crises have not been at the forefront of multilateral security agendas, and, if present, the plans put in place have not worked in practice.[3] This pandemic is an opportunity to change the dialogue surrounding national security priorities and to re-assess the distribution of resources accordingly. Our imminent priorities must equally be: tackling climate change, lifting developing countries out of poverty, and treating future health crises as security issues.

Blending old lessons with new approaches

Firstly, this chapter will look at the way in which leading states have receded from global multilateral security structures and the significant detriment this has had to global security as a whole. Secondly, we will turn to a consideration of how certain multilateral organizations, which in the last four years have encountered significant operational obstacles, might be reinvigorated.[4] To ensure this, there must be general goodwill, along with the desire for genuine, non-transactional partnerships among like-minded states. Thirdly, and lastly, this chapter will turn to an example in which multilateralism is not only challenging but often lacking altogether. Northeast Asian multilateralism is an opportunity to open channels of effective communication between China, North Korea, and Japan. It is a chance to tackle some of that area's traditional security concerns, and could in turn lead to partnerships in addressing and combatting new security challenges. This will aid in strengthening ties and cooperation between these countries, resulting in the establishment of a working structure to tackle those larger issues addressed at the beginning of this paper. We will use the OSCE as an example and guide to how this may be brought about. The chapter will conclude by focusing on the future and on the way in which the latter two sections can contribute to a security landscape with a common, unified purpose: tackling the non-traditional security threats of health crises, rising poverty, and climate change. The below example, detailing the Pacific Islands Forum's (PIF) successes in tackling non-traditional security threats, demonstrates that this is possible.

Regaining leadership and direction

It is not enough to advocate for a shift in the understanding of security if our multilateral organizations are not effectively supported. While there are undoubtedly longstanding and well-working multilateral institutions, large-scale multilateral cooperation has faced numerous unprecedented challenges in recent years. The retreat of various leading powers from international multilateral institutions has constituted a body blow to multilateralism at large, leading to a general movement away from multilateral systems and a stagnation of international security cooperation. Russia's suspension of its participation in the Treaty on Conventional Armed Forces in Europe (CFE) in 2015,[5] following its annexation of the Crimea, The United Kingdom's exit from the European Union in 2020,[6] and the United States' withdrawal from the Joint Comprehensive Plan of Action (JCPOA) (2018),[7] Paris Agreement (2017),[8] Intermediate-Range Nuclear Forces Treaty (INF) (2019),[9] and Open Skies Treaty (2020)[10] have set a worrying trend for the future of multilateral diplomacy. "In the conduct of foreign policy, and especially in times of crisis, a nation's word is its most valuable asset. By pulling out of treaty after treaty, reneging on policy after policy, walking away from US responsibilities, and lying about matters big and small, Trump has bankrupted the United States' word in the world."[11] Diplomacy requires credibility, engagement, and commitment to treaties and organizations based on mutual collaboration. This can only happen if states remain committed to their multilateral security obligations. And this does not solely rest on the United States. All states have a responsibility to uphold those commitments and to ensure a global sense of solidarity and cooperation in the face of apathy and isolationism.

The current trend of non-participation in these multilateral organizations sees inaction and a lack of commitment from nations that would otherwise follow the traditional leaders of the international community. The current insistence by some[12] on labeling the COVID-19 virus the "Wuhan virus," or "Chinese virus" in the face of generating collective, constructive action, is an obvious sign to other major powers that they too could act selfishly; "signaling ... that this emergency ... [is] yet another vehicle for competition rather than coordination."[13] It is clear that non-participation at any meaningful level is detrimental to the global multilateral effort in general, which has found itself without a clear consensus. If the world's traditional multilateral leaders are unwilling to cooperate, leaving an absence of strong political will and economic capital, this leaves very little incentive for anyone else to do so. Therefore, the global post-COVID-19 approach must be to improve relations, rebuild bridges, and regain trust. Absent states must re-engage meaningfully on a global multilateral scale and work to strengthen the international security landscape in its entirety. Our global multilateral systems must be reinvigorated, with the goal that with renewed commitment will come renewed action. Further than this, in recognition that strong global leadership is required to enable action and commitment, traditional partners must once again take up a leadership position. Now is the time to consider and re-evaluate our collective global trajectory and what is important going forward. Now is the time for a new spirit of multilateralism.

A reinvigoration of multilateral security

The Pacific Islands Forum (PIF): An example to follow

The broader significance of the Northeast Asian example is that it sheds light on the importance of regional multilateral forums, which can often do more than much bigger and more disparate ones such as the UN. Pacific Islands Forum (PIF) is an example of an effective non-traditional regional multilateral forum, demonstrating the benefits of unified purpose and a coherent voice. Though they have no significant traditional security concerns, the PIF's (2018) Boe Declaration calls for an expanded concept of security, including "human security, humanitarian assistance, prioritizing environmental security, and regional cooperation in building resilience to disasters and climate change."[14] The Pacific Islands find themselves at the sharp end of the climate crisis. This unified purpose (regarding, among mounting calamitous problems, catastrophic rising sea levels, ocean acidification, and mass forced displacement[15]) has rendered them highly cooperative and effective. They have banded together to implement policies within the PIF region and to advocate for more stringent climate policy reforms globally.[16] And the Pacific Small Islands Developing States (PSIDS) grouping champions their collective interests: "Pacific Island countries have been voting as a bloc, organizing themselves to take on global responsibilities, placing PSIDS candidates in selected international positions, and actively participating in global negotiations."[17] PIF is an example of a multilateral security organization that has broadened its security remit, whose shared goals and imminent dangers enable its member states to commit equally and whose cultural similarities enable effective communication. Their example ought to be emulated on a global scale. The following section sets out such a framework.

The next steps – From absence to cooperation, within three existing frameworks: The UN, NATO, and the OSCE

Broadening the security remit

UN

For the United Nations Security Council (UNSC) to play a role in coordinating responses to public health crises is not unprecedented. The Security Council Resolution 2177 (2014) declared the Ebola outbreak in West Africa a threat to international peace and security.[18] And more recently, the UN's 2030 Agenda and the Sustainable Development Goals (SDGs) have at their core "the link between peace, security and development ... acknowledging the interconnectedness between the drivers of poverty and conflict."[19]

NATO

When the USSR collapsed in 1991, NATO's mission continued; it remained relevant by shifting its focus. As the most robust, interoperable military alliance in the world, NATO has the opportunity to take the lead in re-imaging what security will look like post-COVID-19, and furthermore in finding the means by which it can be useful in non-traditional security settings.

OSCE

At the OSCE's 11th Ministerial Council in 2003, in light of the changing security landscape post 9/11, OSCE Ministers adopted (i) a Strategy to Address Threats to Security and Stability in the Twenty-First Century and (ii) a Strategy Document for the Economic and Environmental Dimension. The latter was "based on an assessment of … existing threats to security in these fields."[20] The authors recommend that a similar forum be held to determine the way forward post COVID-19.

Collaboration and commitment

The success of the above multilateral security institutions, and multilateralism in general, rests on a real will from member states to make these organizations work, to overcome small quarrels in the face of the larger picture.

UN

"The United Nations and its agencies can be important tools in the fight, but they will be only as effective as their powerful members allow them to be."[21]

As noted above, thinking of health crises within a security framework is not without precedent. Bearing in mind UNSC Resolution 2177, the global nature of this current outbreak "makes an even stronger claim for such action."[22] However, partisanship and squabbling within the UNSC, described as a "shambolic disunity,"[23] has made such action not yet possible. The only UN body empowered to authorize military and economic coercion to back its demands,[24] the UNSC has so far failed to adopt a Resolution directed at addressing COVID-19.[25] The severe lack of cooperation from UNSC members, in particular the permanent members, fundamentally calls into question the nature and purpose of the UNSC. Given the unprecedented scale of this pandemic, it is astounding that the UNSC has failed to act in the way that it did with the Ebola crisis in 2014. Nevertheless, despite this unjustifiable delay, the situation is not unsalvageable. There is still time in the coming months for the UNSC to come to an agreement and to take the concrete steps necessary for action to be taken.

NATO

The quality of the NATO alliance largely depends on the amount (or lack thereof) of political consensus among its Heads of State. This fragmented structure affects overall security coordination, strategic direction, and political will to consult and act fast in a crisis.

NATO's inability to act quickly during the COVID-19 crisis speaks to two issues. First, that it does not regard health crises such as pandemics as security issues per se and, second, that NATO members do not think to use NATO in this way. For NATO to become more effective, it needs to be present in the minds of its members. An example to highlight this is the Euro-Atlantic Disaster Response Coordination Centre (EADRCC). While this plays an important role in the coordination of medical and logistical supplies to NATO member states struggling with COVID-19,[26] its assistance needs to be requested by member states. Therefore, for the crisis response arm of NATO to become more efficient, the EARDCC needs to be utilized more effectively.

Ongoing disagreement over NATO burden-sharing has stymied US participation in regional security cooperation. And while one positive outcome of the December 2019 NATO Leaders' meeting was a degree of consensus regarding the 2% spending target, this may now be set back in the post-COVID-19 economic climate. The anticipated catastrophic global recession[27] will likely "oblige national governments to reprioritize their domestic policies and resources, focus their energies on mitigating the fall-out of a severe global economic recession and strengthening their resilience against future shocks."[28] Member states will likely begin to look inward, focusing on recovery rather than meeting their spending commitments. Furthermore, "political and public support for defence spending will be much harder to gain in the future,"[29] as this "small but highly politicised part of the budget"[30] becomes de-prioritized. Yet "the alliance transcends dollars and cents."[31] NATO Member States' commitment is by no means transactional but sacrosanct. NATO is at the very core of the West's national security; "it is the bulwark of the liberal democratic ideal – an alliance of values, which makes it far more durable, reliable, and powerful than partnerships built by coercion or cash."[32] It would thus benefit multilateralism for all NATO Member States to recognize the strategic security interests in the region and continue to uphold their commitment to NATO in the face of a likely spending deficit and economic downturn (Hathaway, 2020). While some states may fail to meet their spending targets, the strength of the alliance extends far beyond this.

OSCE

In its origination as "a multilateral conference for dialogue on Cold War security issues," the OSCE has developed a strong record of relationship management.[33] Its ability to "foster frequent and open-ended communication" stems from its "regular, alliance-free, inclusive and free-ranging dialogue."[34] Such is the centrality of multilateral communication to the OSCE that it has been criticized for being "all words and not enough action."[35] Nevertheless, there are valuable lessons in this approach. In the absence of military capacity (as in NATO) or significant legal capacity (as in the European Union), the OSCE has developed conflict prevention mechanisms by means of frequent, "open dialogue and consensus."[36] "[T]he OSCE's confidence-building activities, combined with its role as a forum for interstate dialogue explicitly linking security with international norms ... fosters a 'propensity to trust' upon which member states are increasingly seeking to give each other the benefit of the doubt."[37] Therefore, the OSCE's efficacy lies in its strength of strategic collaborative discourse across fifty-seven states.

Communication and transparency – The latent multilateral multiplier

Meeting frequently is crucial for effective communication and collaboration. Face-to-face meetings are by far the most effective; however, this is not always possible, and the possibility of in-person meetings will become more uncertain in the wake of COVID-19. High-level person-to-person connections are also essential for maintaining trust and open communication.

UN

Due to the COVID-19 pandemic, the UNSC has not convened a meeting at its New York headquarters since mid-March.[38] While virtual meetings via video conferencing have taken place, this has significantly "[hampered] the kind of person-to-person contact that shapes international diplomacy."[39] Given the highly likely move to greater use of virtual technologies in the future, the UNSC (and most likely all multilateral bodies) must bear in mind the importance of in-person communication and find ways to mitigate its loss.

NATO

On April 2, 2020, NATO held its first virtual Foreign Ministerial Meeting. Though the World Health Organization had declared a pandemic on March 11,[40] it was not until this meeting that NATO consolidated its approach and messaging regarding COVID-19: (i) that it was ready to defend, (ii) that it was ready to coordinate help during the COVID-19 pandemic, and (iii) warning against disinformation campaigns.[41] This speaks to the efficiency and effectiveness of regular meetings and demonstrates that NATO is capable of adapting to the current situation and rising to an unprecedented challenge.

OSCE

The weekly meetings of OSCE's Forum for Security Cooperation (FSC) enable rotating chairmanship by all OSCE members (rotating about every four months). Even relatively small countries, such as Andorra, have been effective in chairing the FSC through this structure. This enables a flat structure that largely guards against a one-size-fits-all mindset. This structure is particularly suited for a relook as it blends military and political advisors but remains largely focused on traditional security concerns such as arms control.

An opportunity for a Northeast Asian security structure

Why this is important?

This chapter has so far outlined elements on which multilateral organizations ought to stop focusing and those to which they ought to turn their attention. It has then outlined three broad factors that would make multilateral organizations more effective: they cannot shift their focus if they do not have a clear remit or if they are unproductive with regard to new definitions of security threats. Now, the chapter will turn to Northeast Asia, where there is currently no overarching multilateral mechanism – in fact, one could argue no mechanism at all – for security cooperation. The 2003 Six Party Talks were thought at the time to be the vehicle to achieve this; however, the hoped-for outcomes have not been realized.[42]

There is a geopolitical area in which traditional security issues have yet to be resolved. While the authors remain steadfast in the argument that these threats pose a comparatively smaller threat than climate change, health crises, and pandemics, they must nevertheless be resolved (or at least, effective communication and collaborative channels must be established) in order to enable broader collaboration in the face of these more pressing threats. North Korea's recent weapons tests,[43] along with China's initial attempts to cover up the significance of the virus during outset of the COVID-19 pandemic,[44] are all the more reason for this to happen *now*, before tensions further escalate and relationships further deteriorate. Thus, we recommend the creation of a Northeast Asian Security Forum as a means by which these tensions might go some way toward being resolved. This subregion of East Asia is a security complex of its own but lacks a fully-fledged institutionalized forum for discussing security concerns. It takes a concerted decision collectively to convene a process that would carve out a security structure. The reality is that there has not been either the political will of the main interlocutors to start such a process or the resources devoted to pushing an idea forward. Nevertheless, the task of strengthening constructive engagement among the countries of East Asia is especially timely and important. Today, Northeast Asia is overdue for a deepened regional security cooperation that would ultimately complement the push toward a redefinition of urgent security threats.

OSCE's role in assisting this structure

The OSCE is now and has been actively engaged in outreach. An important element of the OSCE's ongoing work is to seek to share its experiences with other regions and organizations. The OSCE's ongoing relationship with its Asian and Mediterranean Partners for Co-operation[45] has provided the opportunity to exchange views and knowledge. The Asian Partners include Afghanistan, Australia, Japan, the Republic of Korea, and Thailand. This could, and should, extend to the Northeast Asian region once again and to a greater degree.

Why should the OSCE experience in cooperative security and conflict prevention be of interest to the region? First of all, the authors recognize that the historical conditions that produced the OSCE are quite different from those that prevail in Northeast or East Asia today. The end of the Cold War and even the events of September 11, 2001, have affected the OSCE region and particularly Northeast Asia differently. However, there are elements of the OSCE experience that are of practical value in certain parts of this diverse region.

The previously mentioned FSC offers an example of a cooperative security body that could be tailored for application in Asia, particularly Northeast Asia, filling the need for a regional multilateral security mechanism that mixes military and political advisors. As a permanent standing body it meets weekly and has dedicated delegation representatives who can engage in the detailed bilateral or multilateral negotiations often needed for forward movement. The FSC negotiates Confidence and Security Building Measures (CSBMs), an instrument that is lacking in Northeast Asia and oversees their implementation. One cannot start with CSBMs without placing them, however ambitious and admirable, into first a workable institutional structure for a dialogue that can address current and underlying political challenges to peace and security within the region. Nevertheless, such CSBMs would ultimately provide a basis to address the new threats detailed at the outset of the chapter – health crises, rising poverty, and climate change.

Although the potential of the FSC can only serve as a model, it is one that the decision makers framing the debate on East Asian and Northeast Asian security structures need to carefully consider; similar work has already been done within a geographic area that comprises fifty-seven countries. The Forum, like all other bodies in the OSCE, is a consensus-driven body. That naturally restricts what any single country can accomplish, especially considering the range of views held in an organization of so many members. Yet, the FSC and OSCE offer a working regional venue for its participating States to discuss – in an open forum or in smaller groups – issues of national interest. That fact, in and of itself, is an invaluable confidence- and security-building measure. Finally, as a result of a supporting Secretariat, the rotating Chairmanships, and the Troika that bridges past and incoming Chairs, the FSC has managed to include and address with deliverable results some key emerging traditional security interests.

This brief synopsis provides some idea of what the FSC is and does. Given the sophistication of most countries of Northeast Asia, the subregion has the capability to establish an institutionalized set of cooperative security measures or CSBMs along the lines of those negotiated by the FSC/OSCE. If the countries of the subregion have the political will and the desire, the FSC and broader OSCE would certainly be able to take COVID-19 as an impetus to share more with regional states on practices appropriate for the region – and in clear regard for Northeast Asia, which lacks many such measures.

The challenge of introducing the OSCE's experience in political-military confidence-building within the Asian region consists of more than simply finding the right workable content for individual measures. It is a more fundamental problem given the doggedly complex political impasse within which any such regional initiative would have to be discharged. It rests with the ability to overcome a pervading win-lose perception: the perception that negotiating even minimalist but mutually supportive security measures would somehow create a disproportionate "benefit" for some parties and a perceived and corresponding "deficit" for one's own strategic and political role in the region. It is hopeful that, "[a]s a global governance practice characterized by an inclusive, institutionalized, and principled form of dialog, the multilateral procedure generates a number of processual benefits - mutually recognizable patterns of action, typically moderate solutions, and legitimate policies whose large ownership eases their effective implementation - which, taken together, strengthen the political impetus for global cooperation, regardless of the policies adopted."[46] "The move from purely interest-based behaviour towards commonly respected principles should over time lead to increasing trust among actors."[47] Yet this also requires political and cooperative will. The driving force must be a broad political endorsement to engage actively in this process to then address these new concerns of health crises, rising poverty, and climate change. This is, in historical terms, agreement among the countries in Northeast Asia, plus traditional partners such as the European Union and the United States, to make a "Helsinki"[48] commitment for Northeast Asia. The creation of a Northeast Asian multilateral entity, then, is an area where the OSCE, due to its already established framework, could materially help multilateralism if politically endorsed.

Conclusion

Focus on traditional security issues is a ready-made distraction from those that pose a much greater threat in the post-COVID-19 global setting. There is a very real sense in which these traditional security mechanisms are self-sustaining and not only distract from the greater issues but produce the very issues they purport to protect against. Securitized migration has created more, and more dangerous, migrant routes, creating an escalating sense of crisis and thereby justifying more resources being poured in to combat it – and to continue the cycle.[49] Countries at the forefront of disarmament talks continue to be the largest arms suppliers in the world.[50] Focus on traditional security is not only overly prioritized, but it is a dangerous distraction from future threats. There is time to combat, and mitigate, these disparities. But that window is closing fast. And to do this effectively, it is not sufficient simply to shift our security focus. We must reinvigorate our international multilateral security organizations such as NATO, the OSCE, and the UN. These have been too often marginalized in the global withdrawal from multilateral cooperation. Traditional leaders refuse to lead, and what's more, have absented themselves from some of the most significant multilateral security successes of the 21st century. In order for there to be a shift in the importance and focus of security and its nexus with emerging threats, the absent leaders must once more participate on the international stage – and must take on a united position that no single state has succeeded in filling. These multilateral structures, and the states that make them up, must make concerted efforts to improve their collaboration and commitment and communication. It is only by doing this, and repairing the damage that has been done over the last several years, that we may hope to be effective in combating the coming crises, the scale and destruction of which we have never before seen. In this vein, the authors see an opportunity, long-overlooked but increasingly pressing as the scale of international crises deepen, for a Northeast Asian multilateral security structure. The tensions between China, North Korea, and Japan are untenable, and unsustainable. It is only by instituting a multilateral structure and opening channels of communication and cooperation that these states may come together and address their geopolitical security issues. It is not until the traditional security threats are resolved (or at least engaged in dialogue) that they may then turn, now in collaboration, to the larger problems of health crises, rising poverty, and climate change which the authors consider a now higher priority.

Notes

1. The views in this chapter are solely those of the authors and do not represent the opinions of current or past organizations.
2. Tony Blair Institute for Global Change. (2020) "How extremist groups are responding to Covid-19."
3. Pandemic preparedness has been focused overwhelmingly on pandemic influenza rather than a coronavirus-related pandemic. See, for example, World Health Organization. (2017) "Pandemic influenza risk management." See also Davies, S. (2013) "National security and pandemics." UN Chronicle. On the difficulties of states in building pandemic preparedness capacities, especially in the face of already-struggling health systems.
4. Deeper, D. (2019) "Emmanuel Macron warns Europe: NATO is becoming brain-dead." The Economist.
5. Reif, K. (2015) "Russia completes CFE Treaty suspension." Arms Control Today. Arms Control Association.
6. Barnes, P. (2020) "Brexit: what happens now?" BBC News.
7. Nephew, R. (2018) "The US withdrawal from the JCPOA: what to look out for over the next year." Center on Global Energy Policy, Columbia School of International and Public Affairs.
8. Pompeo, M. (2019) "On the U.S. withdrawal from the Paris Agreement." U.S. Department of State.
9. Gramer, R. and Seligman, L. (2019) "The INF treaty is dead. Is new START next?." Foreign Policy.
10. Reif, K. and Bugos, S. (2020) "U.S. to withdraw from Open Skies Treaty." *Arms Control Today*. Arms Control Association.
11. Biden, J. (2020) "Why America must lead again." Foreign Affairs.
12. Graziosi, G. (2020) "Coronavirus: Mike Pompeo insists G7 use 'Wuhan Virus' – but world officials refuse." Independent.
13. Power, S. (2020) "This won't end for anyone until it ends for everyone." The New York Times.
14. Pacific Islands Forum Secretariat. (2018) "Boe Declaration on regional security."
15. Ackman, M., Naupa, A. and Tuimalealiifano, P. (2018) "Boe Declaration: navigating an uncertain Pacific." The Interpreter. The Lowy Institute.

16. Alam, Mayaz et al. "Strategic re-engagement: advancing U.S. leadership in multilateral diplomacy." Institute for the Study of Diplomacy. May 2020.
17. Beck, C. (2020) "Geopolitics of the Pacific Islands: how should the Pacific Islands States advance their strategic and security interests?" Security Challenges, vol. 16, no. 1, pp. 11–16.
18. United Nations Security Council, Resolution 2177. (2014).
19. Ackman, M., Naupa, A. and Tuimalealiifano, P. (2018) "Boe Declaration: navigating an uncertain Pacific." The Interpreter. The Lowy Institute.
20. 11th Ministerial Council. (2003). Organization for Security And Co-operation in Europe.
21. Power, S. (2020) "This won't end for anyone until it ends for everyone." The New York Times.
22. Yang, L. (2020) "The Coronavirus requires international security cooperation." Carnegie-Tsinghua Center for Global Policy.
23. Gladstone, R. (2020) "U.N. Security Council 'Missing In Action' in Coronavirus fight." The New York Times.
24. Gladstone, R. (2020) "U.N. Security Council 'Missing In Action' in Coronavirus fight." The New York Times.
25. United Nations Security Council. "Resolutions adopted by the Security Council in 2020."
26. Transatlantic Security Jam. (2020).
27. Elliot, L. (2020) "Prepare for the coronavirus global recession." The Guardian.
28. Transatlantic Security Jam. (2020).
29. Transatlantic Security Jam. (2020).
30. Tocci, N. (2020) "COVID-19 and its impact on Euro Atlantic Security." Covid-19: The Policy Response. London School of Economics and Political Science.
31. Biden, J. (2020) "Why America must lead again." Foreign Affairs.
32. Biden, J. (2020) "Why America must lead again." Foreign Affairs.
33. Berzins, C. A. (2004) The puzzle of trust in international relations: risk and relationship management in the Organization for Security and Cooperation in Europe, p. 184.
34. Berzins, C. A. (2004). The puzzle of trust in international relations: risk and relationship management in the Organization for Security and Cooperation in Europe, p. 184.
35. Berzins, C. A. (2004). The puzzle of trust in international relations: risk and relationship management in the Organization For Security and Cooperation in Europe, p. 196.
36. Berzins, C. A. (2004). The puzzle of trust in international relations: risk and relationship management in the Organization For Security and Cooperation in Europe, p. 183.
37. Berzins, C. A. (2004). The puzzle of trust in international relations: risk and relationship management in the Organization For Security and Cooperation in Europe, p. 2.
38. Gladstone, R. (2020) "U.N. Security Council 'Missing In Action' in Coronavirus fight." The New York Times.
39. Gladstone, R. (2020) "U.N. Security Council 'Missing In Action' in Coronavirus fight." The New York Times.
40. World Health Organization Newsroom. (2020) "WHO Timeline – Covid-19." World Health Organization.
41. North Atlantic Treaty Organization. (2020) "Declarations by NATO Foreign Ministers."
42. Bajoria, J. and Xu, B. (2013) "The Six Party Talks on North Korea's nuclear program." Council on Foreign Relations.

43. Sang-Hun, C. (2020) "North Korea launches two short-range ballistic missiles." The New York Times.
44. Davidson, H. (2020) "First Covid-19 case happened in November, China government records show – report." The Guardian.
45. Organization for Security and Co-Operation in Europe. "Partners for co-operation."
46. Pouliot, V. (2011) "Multilateralism as an end in itself." International Studies Perspectives, vol. 12, no. 1, pp. 18–26.
47. Jokela, J. (2011) "Global Governance and effective multilateralism." European Union Institute for Security Studies (EUISS), pp. 51–60. The G-20: A pathway to effective multilateralism?
48. The Editors of Encyclopaedia Britannica. (2019) "Helsinki Accords." Encyclopædia Britannica, Inc.: Encyclopædia Britannica.
49. Andersson, R. (2016) "Europe's failed 'fight' against irregular migration: ethnographic notes on a counterproductive industry." Journal of Ethnic and Migration Studies, vol. 42, no. 7.
50. For example, China, Russia, South Korea, Turkey, and the United States are significant suppliers. See Stockholm International Peace Research Institute. (2020) "SIPRI Arms Transfers Database."

References

Ackman, M., Naupa, A. and Tuimalealiifano, P. (2018) "Boe Declaration: navigating an uncertain Pacific." The Interpreter. The Lowy Institute. Retrieved on May 22 2020 from https://www.lowyinstitute.org/the-interpreter/boe-declaration-navigating-uncertain-pacific

Andersson, R. (2016) "Europe's failed 'fight' against irregular migration: ethnographic notes on a counterproductive industry." *Journal of Ethnic and Migration Studies*, vol. 42, no. 7, Retrieved on 20 June 2020 from https://www.tandfonline.com/doi/full/10.1080/1369183X.2016.1139446

Bajoria, J. and Xu, B. (2013) "The six party talks on North Korea's nuclear program." *Council on Foreign Relations*. Retrieved on 25 June 2020 from https://www.cfr.org/backgrounder/six-party-talks-north-koreas-nuclear-program

Barnes, P. (2020) "Brexit: what happens now?" *BBC News*. Retrieved on 23 June 2020 from https://www.bbc.co.uk/news/uk-politics-46393399

Beck, C. (2020) "Geopolitics of the Pacific Islands: how should the Pacific Islands States advance their strategic and security interests?" *Security Challenges*, vol. 16, no. 1, pp. 11–16. Retrieved on 22 May 2020 from https://www.jstor.org/stable/pdf/26908762.pdf?ab_segments=0%25252Fbasic_SYC-5152%25252Fcontrol&refreqid=excelsior%253A1b9a26e24a91da65973b15fe9ef264ff

Berzins, C. A. (2004). *The Puzzle of Trust in International Relations: Risk and Relationship Management in the Organization for Security and Cooperation in Europe*. PhD thesis, London School of Economics and Political Science (United Kingdom). Retrieved on 20 June 2020 from http://etheses.lse.ac.uk/1741/

Biden, J. (2020) "Why America must lead again." *Foreign Affairs*. Retrieved on 22 May 2020 from https://www.foreignaffairs.com/articles/united-states/2020-01-23/why-america-must-lead-again

Davidson, H. (2020) "First Covid-19 case happened in November, China government records show – report." *The Guardian*. Retrieved on 30 June 2020 from https://www.theguardian.com/world/2020/mar/13/first-covid-19-case-happened-in-november-china-government-records-show-report

Davies, S. (2013) "National security and pandemics." *UN Chronicle*. Retrieved on 24 June 2020 from https://www.un.org/en/chronicle/article/national-security-and-pandemics

Deeper, D. (2019) "Emmanuel Macron warns Europe: NATO is becoming brain-dead." *The Economist*. Retrieved on 20 June 2020 from https://www.economist.com/europe/2019/11/07/emmanuel-macron-warns-europe-nato-is-becoming-brain-dead

Dworkin, A. and Gowan, R. (2019) "Rescuing multilateralism." *European Council on Foreign Relations*. Retrieved on 22 May 2020 from https://www.jstor.org/stable/pdf/resrep21495.pdf?ab_segments=0%25252Fbasic_SYC-5152%25252Fcontrol&refreqid=excelsior%253A7cbe6a32f1459611235fcaedf27681b7

Elliot, L. (2020) "Prepare for the coronavirus global recession." *The Guardian*. Retrieved on 20 June 2020 from https://www.theguardian.com/business/2020/mar/15/prepare-for-the-coronavirus-global-recession

Gladstone, R. (2020) "U.N. Security Council 'Missing In Action' in Coronavirus fight." *The New York Times*. Retrieved on 22 May 2020 from https://www.nytimes.com/2020/04/02/world/americas/coronavirus-united-nations-guterres.html?searchResultPosition=1

Gramer, R. and Seligman, L. (2019) "The INF Treaty is dead. Is new START next?." *Foreign Policy*. Retrieved on 30 June 2020 from https://foreignpolicy.com/2019/02/01/the-inf-treaty-is-dead-is-new-start-next-russia-arms/.

Graziosi, G. (2020) "Coronavirus: Mike Pompeo insists G7 use 'Wuhan Virus' – but world officials refuse." *Independent*. Retrieved on 20 June 2020 from https://www.independent.co.uk/news/coronavirus-g7-wuhan-virus-mike-pompeo-trump-a9426261.html

Hathaway, O. (2020) "COVID-19 shows how the U.S. got national security wrong." *Just Security*. Retrieved on 22 May 2020 from https://www.justsecurity.org/69563/covid-19-shows-how-the-u-s-got-national-security-wrong

Jokela, J. (2011) "Global governance and effective multilateralism." *European Union Institute for Security Studies (EUISS)*, pp. 51–60. The G-20: a pathway to effective multilateralism? Retrieved on 22 May 2020 from https://www.jstor.org/stable/pdf/resrep07003.7.pdf?ab_segments=0%25252Fbasic_SYC-5152%25252Fcontrol&refreqid=excelsior%253A42c3904f383f1d68fd6207316e829fb7

Nephew, R. (2018) "The US withdrawal from the JCPOA: what to look out for over the next year." *Center on Global Energy Policy, Columbia School of International and Public Affairs*. Retrieved on 30 June 2020 from https://energypolicy.columbia.edu/research/commentary/us-withdrawal-jcpoa-what-look-out-over-next-year

North Atlantic Treaty Organization. (2020) "Declarations by NATO foreign ministers." Retrieved on 25 June 2020 from https://www.nato.int/cps/en/natohq/official_texts_174855.htm?selectedLocale=en

Organization for Security and Co-operation in Europe. "Partners for co-operation." Retrieved on 25 June 2020 from https://www.osce.org/partners-for-cooperation

Pacific Islands Forum Secretariat. (2018) "Boe Declaration on regional security." Retrieved on 22 May 2020 from https://www.forumsec.org/boe-declaration-on-regional-security

Pompeo, M. (2019) "On the U.S. withdrawal from the Paris Agreement." U.S. Department of State. Retrieved on 30 June 2020 from https://www.state.gov/on-the-u-s-withdrawal-from-the-paris-agreement/

Pouliot, V. (2011) "Multilateralism as an end in itself." *International Studies Perspectives*, vol. 12, no. 1, pp. 18–26. Retrieved on 22 May 2020 from https://www.jstor.org/stable/pdf/44218646.pdf?ab_segments=0%252Fbasic_SYC-5152%252Fcontrol&refreqid=excelsior%3A7147f94b7cfb9e5a9abfa6e853fbcdb6

Power, S. (2020) "This won't end for anyone until it ends for everyone." *The New York Times.* Retrieved on 22 May 2020 from https://www.nytimes.com/2020/04/07/opinion/coronavirus-united-states-leadership.html

Reif, K. (2015) "Russia completes CFE Treaty suspension." *Arms Control Today.* Arms Control Association. Retrieved on 20 June 2020 from https://www.armscontrol.org/act/2015-04/news-briefs/russia-completes-cfe-treaty-suspension

Reif, K. and Bugos, S. (2020) "U.S. to withdraw from Open Skies Treaty." *Arms Control Today.* Arms Control Association. Retrieved on 30 June 2020 from https://www.armscontrol.org/act/2020-06/news/us-withdraw-open-skies-treaty

Sang-Hun, C. (2020) "North Korea launches two short-range ballistic missiles." *The New York Times.* Retrieved on 22 May 2020 from https://www.nytimes.com/2020/03/28/world/asia/north-korea-missile-launch.html

Stockholm International Peace Research Institute. (2020) "SIPRI arms transfers database." Retrieved on 25 June 2020 from https://www.sipri.org/databases/armstransfers

The Editors of Encyclopædia Britannica. (2019) "Helsinki accords." Encyclopædia Britannica, Inc.: Encyclopædia Britannica. Retrieved on 30 June 2020 from https://www.britannica.com/event/Helsinki-Accords

Tocci, N. (2020) "COVID-19 and its impact on Euro Atlantic Security." Covid-19: The Policy Response. London School of Economics and Political Science. Retrieved on 22 May 2020 from https://www.facebook.com/lseps/videos/1579936925515388/

Tony Blair Institute for Global Change. (2020) "How extremist groups are responding to Covid-19." Retrieved on 22 May 2020 from https://institute.global/policy/snapshot-how-extremist-groups-are-responding-covid-19-6-may-2020

Transatlantic Security Jam. (2020). Securing the Post COVID-19 Future. Retrieved on 22 May 2020 from https://www.collaborationjam.com/j5/3964235/#/postJam

United Nations Security Council. "Resolutions adopted by the Security Council in 2020." Retrieved on 20 June 2020 from https://www.un.org/securitycouncil/content/resolutions-adopted-security-council-2020

United Nations Security Council, Resolution 2177. (2014). Retrieved on 22 May 2020 from http://unscr.com/en/resolutions/doc/2177

World Health Organization. (2017) "Pandemic influenza risk management." Retrieved on 24 June 2020 from https://apps.who.int/iris/bitstream/handle/10665/259893/WHO-WHE-IHM-GIP-2017.1-eng.pdf?sequence=1

World Health Organization Newsroom. (2020) "WHO Timeline – Covid-19." *World Health Organization.* Retrieved on 25 June 2020 from https://www.who.int/news-room/detail/27-04-2020-who-timeline—covid-19

Yang, L. (2020) "The coronavirus requires international security cooperation." *Carnegie-Tsinghua Center for Global Policy.* Retrieved on 22 May 2020 from https://carnegietsinghua.org/2020/04/07/coronavirus-requires-international-security-cooperation-pub-81482

11th Ministerial Council. (2003). Organization for Security and Co-operation in Europe. Retrieved on 20 June 2020 from https://www.osce.org/event/mc_2003

5 Health economic model for developing countries to combat pandemics

Chandra Nilanga Samarasinghe

Introduction

The COVID-19 pandemic is not just a disaster; it has taught many lessons to people to think about the social and economic norms of modern civilization, the pros, and cons of globalization, the importance of developing as a whole (population within the country and globally as well). Lessons of equality and equity and questions on the usefulness of sending a rocket to the moon before fulfilling the basic requirements of people have also had to be considered.

Most scholars are of the opinion that the post-pandemic era will not be a continuation of pre-pandemic times. They would like to name the situation "extraordinary" and the post-pandemic era as a "new normal world." The new normal world would consist of two segments,

1 The period until the herd immunity will develop naturally or by a vaccine. This would prolong for at least 18 to 24 months or maybe more. The determining factor of everything is social distancing.
2 The period after the herd immunity develops.
   When the social distancing restrictions are lifted, the world would theoretically not go back to the pre-2020 era. Measures adopted to combat the Corona pandemic that have been proven to be advantageous and economically cost effective will be continued: Work from home, online deals, communication, some leisure activities, gig economic activities, discontinuation of disadvantageous bilateral and international agreements, and the continuation of import substitute productions (if they have won a piece of market and stability due to non-competition during the pandemic). Disadvantageous adaptations will be given up and reverted to 2019.

Indeed, the real new normal world is going to be the interaction between society and the economically cost-effective adaptations that enterprises and governments refuse to abandon even though it has resulted in unemployment, lower earnings, and a widening gap between rich and poor.

If that is the case, the question that developing nations face is, are they going to belong to the new normal world or remain in the old world? We are trying to

DOI: 10.4324/9781003197416-5

explain the scenario faced by developing countries taking Sri Lanka as an example. This is the timely question that Sri Lankans must answer today: Is the island nation ready to take up the challenge which was missed on several occasions since independence and that the Corona epidemic has presented?

Or are you going to be a spectator again? If you are ready, here are the propositions. This is not the first or the last biological or another kind of global disaster the country has faced or is facing. If you have learned the lessons from the previous challenges, you may understand that any disaster will bring the world back to its' very basics.

To introduce social, economic, or any other kind of reform to a country, we have to accept and consider the values of the country – its policies, political willingness, nature and culture of the politics and people, corruption, debts, etc. your suggestions must be adapted to the existing system, not to some hypothetically country born yesterday. Many scholars forget this simple truth when drafting policy recommendations. Countries should count their own experiences as well as foreign ones. Sri Lanka has had good and bad experiences of the closed economy (1970–1977) and open economy since 1977. The exemplary model countries for Sri Lanka should be Rwanda, Nigeria, Mexico, and Hong Kong, not Singapore, South Korea, or a western country with totally different social, cultural, economic, and political values.

I stress again, the strategy for facing an epidemic/disaster absolutely depends on the country's status, namely, economy, social, education, culture, the policy of the current government, qualities of political leaders, government servants, and people.

In the case of Sri Lanka, which recently held general election, an important political event happened soon after the presidential election. It was clear that all the policies and non-political events too were designed around it. If we look at the reality, we should admit that "Election first, Corona and rest thereafter" was the thinking in the country. However, in the hope of a better future, the election was held with maximum safety measures to bring in a stable single-minded government to fight against Corona with a concrete productive policy plan and take the opportunities to rise to the status of a developing country. The people looked to bring in a strong parliament, ensuring policy decisions empowering common people's interests can be taken and the island nation is not divided party-wise in this volatile pandemic period. (This is what the wise people of South Korea have done.)

Indeed, this is the litmus test of President Gotababaya Rajapakshe's first hundred days as it was for the first 100 days of the "Yahaplana" government in 2015. He governs the country as the president, chief of cabinet, and defense forces with his prime minister brother Mahinda, keen party organizer Brother organizer Basil and a bunch of acquittances, and his nominees as cabinet ministers and secretaries and especially with the unconditional support of major ethnoreligious group, Sinhala Buddhists and media, all the key religious leaders and trade unions (unfortunately not the minority ethnic groups). It is a situation where the majority of government officers, academics, technocrats, professionals, and businessmen (Viyath Maga) are his party supporters and loyalists. The Dismantled and weakest-ever opposition party is an extra advantage. What else would you want to battle the Corona pandemic if you have a good plan?

Well-preparedness solves the problem by 50%. There is nothing so practical as a good theory (Senanayaka and Darshana 2019). Hence, our intention is to introduce a sophisticated and workable disaster management plan for any developing country, taking Sri Lanka as an example.

We recommend eight socio-health economic safety nets to be introduced and implemented before, during, and after a disaster. Also, if a country has a similar disaster management plan, we invite them to study our plan, adopt and absorb the parts they may have missed. And if they could contribute some worthy suggestions to enhance our model plan, they are always welcome.

The socio health economic model we suggest here can be implemented not only in pandemics but in the event of other disasters too. As in an earthquake, tsunami, flood, landslide, etc. (on a smaller scale compared to pandemics).

The necessity of a strong disaster management policy

Though every country may have a Disaster Management Act already, we recommend that it must be very strong. One of the biggest lessons taught by the Corona Pandemic is the problem of not having a powerful and comprehensive act ready for implementation.

For each disaster, the prime minister should bring a bill to the parliament to empower the act, e.g. COVID-19 Pandemic Bill. It shall announce an extraordinary situation and executive orders to mitigate and control the disaster.

It shall call for an action plan from local authorities with a budget, time frame, and timely calculated results (mileposts). If 50% of the workload of the action plan is unable to be fulfilled by the local body at the milepost of 60%, the task will be transferred to the central government. The central government agencies in the local body shall inform of the progress of the task to the central government and it should design the disaster management plan with a time frame at the milepost of 40% while studying the errors of the local plan.

If both institutes are not able to complete the task within the said time frames, they must go to a combined project. 2/3 of responsibility & accountability shall be borne by the local body and 1/3 of responsibility & accountability by the central body.

Pros:

- Responsibility & accountability go to the grass-roots level
- No blame or criticism on the national level politicians over the trials and errors
- National level does the guiding, monitoring, and supervising
- Every citizen is responsible & accountable for disaster management and mitigation (nothing about us without us policy)

- Some critical and important but not attractive decisions could be implemented under local authority shield. The central government could act as a protector and mitigator of internal as well as external (even foreign) pressures on such activities

Cons: No cons

One of the weakest characteristics of local governing bodies is the lack of consultation with resource persons in the sphere of designing or implementing development or any other projects as done at the national level. This should be corrected and brought into practice. Indeed, it is a very important part of democracy.

The biggest lesson we learned from the Corona pandemic was that every government should be ready to supply the basic life needs for the nation under any circumstances before thinking of advanced or luxury lifestyle facilities for the nation. Building basic infrastructure facilities is more important than building the highest towers, the biggest playgrounds, bullet trains, and sending rockets to the moon.

- Compulsory Transport
- Compulsory food supply
- Compulsory medical facilities
- Compulsory infrastructure facilities (water, electricity, gas, internet)

There is a good side to a disaster too.

While maintaining the basic requirements of the community, this will lead to inevitable savings by the middle-class family. (The average saving of a middle-class family in Switzerland during the lockdown period was CHF 2200.00 [McCain, 2015].). No buying of luxurious, not essential foods, sparingly buying clothes and perfumes, etc., delayed buying of non-essential electronic equipment and led to the postponement of or no outings.

Work from home culture

One lesson taught by the pandemic is the restructuring of working style. We learned that some or a significant amount of work could be done from home while attending to the other work of the family with the same or greater efficiency.

Hence, we strongly suggest identifying the Jobs that could be done from home; this should be encouraged with a cap of 60%. Work from home culture will be continued after the pandemic; working from home is not just sitting in front of a computer. It is a short-term culture in a pandemic period but should acquire many additional provisions like home delivery of essential goods, online banking/money activities, health (physical and mental activities), teaching, recreational (leisure) activities, etc.

Delivery of essential foods: Online ordering, paying methods should be established. Liquor and beverages will be distributed in exchange for 20% additional payment (donation) to the Disaster Management Fund (DMF). Ten percent increase of the beverages and cigarettes could be factored in during the period of disaster.

Priority will be given to online customer care services, with special privileges, benefits, and discounts given. Online banking is further encouraged. Online booths/portals should be established in all banks. Many ATMs will be established in secured areas. Police stations, post offices, supermarkets, railway stations, main bus stands, patrol sheds, Assistant Government Agents (AGA) offices, government establishments are places identified for ATM installations. All Public relationship officials will be encouraged to work online at private as well as at public institutes.

Lockdown services

When an area or a country is in lockdown, some auxiliary services have to be supplied to people's doorsteps for example, electricians, plumbers, and other minor services (online services and critical visits must be done).

Domestic health care services for wound care, mental health care, and care for Paraplegics also need to be supplied.

In our Health Economic Model, we suggest eight kinds of safety nets to assure the rational smooth running of the affected community and region.

- Finance net
- Food net
- Health net
- Power net/Administration net
- Education net
- Transport net
- Industries net
- Information net

Finance net

The biggest issue that any country faces when unexpected disasters occur (though some disasters like droughts could be identified and predicted in some vulnerable areas) is that there is insufficient liquid money with the government that it could use in such a situation. All developed countries have reserves of currency and gold that may be sufficient for several years, unlike developing countries.

Therefore, our first proposal is how you can overcome that issue.

- Introducing a DMF.
- In total, 1% from every employee's monthly wage, 2% from every employer, 2% from government.
- Main duty of the fund is securing the basic income of employees during a disaster

- One cent per rupee from every money transaction.
- During the period of disaster, the prices of cigarettes, beverages, wheat flour products (namely buns and pastries), and petrol will be increased by 10% by the government. There will be no increase in the price of bread and other oils.
- Introducing an ATM card that could be used during the disaster period only.
- All citizens are registered at the DMF at birth for benefits.
- All citizens are eligible for benefits without discrimination. Equality & equity is maintained, and the same amount is paid to every citizen which is adequate for essential daily needs.

The same system is applied from the most senior politicians, government servants, and businessmen to daily wage earners and the unemployed too, which will bring you to a time period of true communism/socialism. Hence, all the persons in the affected region suffering from similar financial and social difficulties, and disturbances, will work together and give their maximum contribution to overcoming the crisis quickly.

I will explain this by taking "drought" as a disaster. In an agricultural region, farmers are the backbone, and the main income source of the area and all other services and lifestyles depend on agriculture.

In case of a drought, only the farmers are seriously affected and the other categories like education, administration (because of monthly wages), and businesses (because of undisturbed income) are marginally affected and are likely to suffer less. Therefore, the burden of disaster will not be felt equally by the whole community, and you may see the reaction accordingly (less contribution from less affected categories to get out from the crisis sooner). Equal treatment policy under the disaster management act will make a tremendous change in the attitude of a community to find a solution together.

If we elaborate more taking the North Central Province of Sri Lanka as the affected region, the affected population is not only the farmers but from the governor, chief minister, cabinet ministers, parliament members elected from the region, down to all government officers and businessmen to the unemployed, forest destroyers, Chena cultivators, sand and soil smugglers, and those who indiscriminately use water from the reservoirs. This will influence the teachers, researchers, responsible government officers, policymakers, and politicians to foresee the disasters/crisis to be faced by the community beforehand. Every member of the community takes equal opportunity to bear the responsibility as well as accountability in their own region.

Teaching institutes to teach scientific agriculture. Researchers have to develop crops resistant to drought that consume less water, etc.

Politicians and civil servants have to maintain law and order of the area (no smuggling of soil and sand, water, and water reservoirs are preserved), policymaking, and policy implementation boosting eco-friendly agricultural modern lifestyle in the region.

The fund can be utilized only during a disaster situation, passed by parliament with a 2/3 majority.

If the parliament does not decide on the time, any citizen can go to the supreme court for violation of their fundamental rights.

The Supreme Court can give directions to the government, when, where, to whom, how much, how long with essential steps and guidelines that should solve the situation and correct the errors, mistakes, and wrongdoings of citizens and as well as of the government.

(This will become the biggest social welfare fund of any country within ten years).

Savings during disaster period

Due to the stoppage of non-essential expenses, limited vehicle usage, limited outings, and social events some money will be saved by the people. Special interest rates will be paid for savings during the disaster periods.

One of the biggest issues during a disaster is identifying individuals eligible for financial compensation such as those who are self-employed. Some of the self-employed are part-timers who also have a permanent job or are pensioners. Hence, by paying a standard sum for all the members in affected communities, this method will avoid a person receiving other allowances under different categories.

Donating and collecting goods for affected people is usually a disorganized processes in times of disaster. We suggest establishing a central non-governmental organization so that accountability to the government is ensured.

Economic opportunities

As history reveals, most of the developed countries in the world have progressed bravely and boldly, facing challenges during or after a major crisis like the second world war or internal revolutions.

Some countries had outstripped others by taking great risks when other nations were afraid to take up.

Vasco de Gama, Columbus, and other great explorers and sailors brought their tiny lands to great empires by challenging the odds. The histories of Portugal, Spain, Holland, and Denmark have been rewritten by these intrepid explorers.

The Corona Pandemic first appeared as a health crisis; hence the health economic part of the economy was highlighted and expanded due to the high demand with low or no supply of medicines and equipment to mitigate and control Corona.

A new market is being opened for COVID-19 test kits, polymerase chain reaction (PCR) machines, vaccines, drugs, medical equipment, namely ICU beds, ventilators, hygienic products, face masks, and personal protection kits, and setting up mobile hospitals, instant hospitals, the job market for trained health care professionals, etc. Also, many research opportunities in the health, economic, social, medical fields. Aviation Industry: Charter flights across the world, cargo flights

We encourage the idea of Economic Nationalism if it has high-cost utility value. A global crisis like the Corona Pandemic is an eye-opener for many countries to think of cost-utility instead of cost-effectiveness or cost–benefit. In the new normal world after Corona, it would be the former rather than the latter. But it all depends on the definition of the concept you give.

Also, another economic opportunity has emerged due to the policy of the Trump administration of the United States, Japan, and Korea to shift their industries from Chinese soil over allegations that China concealed the true facts of COVID-19 at the initial state. If a country could provide almost similar facilities as given by China to these industries, it could attract them. Supply of materials, skilled labor, and diligent long working hours (Chinese way) are among the factors required to secure such opportunities.

Job-hunting agencies

Many immigrants are losing their jobs during the pandemic. Many who have been engaged in unskilled and semiskilled jobs would not be able to return to their jobs after the endemic having gone back to their own countries. If our recruiting agencies stay ready to find them and provide essential training and language skills, we can make use of their skills before the rest of the world.

Global Disasters encourage working together rather than in isolation even though the movements have been restricted. Sharing information, knowledge, technology, resources even financial assistance will synergize your ability to face the disaster. Therefore, dreaming for complete autarky or anything even closer to it is far from mere reality. The deep wounds and later the scars caused by Corona Pandemic may last long. The longer the lockdown/curfew, the deeper the wounds and slower the healing of the economy.

If you closely study the rate of spread, rate of infection, rate of severing from infected cases, and rate of death, they are remarkably and significantly low in developing countries when compared with developed countries. My observation is that most of the developing countries did not understand the advantageous situation they were in and did not take the fair risk of working with COVID-19 from the beginning while the developed countries (Western) are struggling with a high rate of spread, high rate of infection, high rate of severing and high rate of deaths. They were totally trapped by fear and scare spreading and marketing by western media giants, the World Health Organization, and their own health professional bodies. (It is understandable that WHO could not issue revolutionary statements or guidelines for risky proactive recommendations to build the economic status of developing countries because it is a healthy body that has to raise the alarm even in the case of very mild health risks to safeguard itself.)

Given the risks associated with investing in developing countries, we have noticed that investors will withdraw their money invested in stock markets in developing countries and trend to invest in stable western economies though the profit is much less but carries a low risk comparatively while being over-reliant on the US dollars for trade and finance, though the United States and the Trump administration are not attractive. If the central banks of developing countries are smart enough and have plans to confidently recover from the disaster within one or two years, they can give guarantees to the investors with fixed assets to hold them and shut down the stock exchange markets for longer times.

Many scholars of developing countries and some of the developed countries think the economies of both developing and developed countries would fall low after the pandemic and remain the same for years and years. But due to reserves of currency and gold, rich countries will stand despite everything against them in a short period. Indeed what could happen is, by purchasing assets of developing countries and their central banks and providing low-interest loans with grace periods to maintain the liquidity that will prevent the collapse of *economies* of the third world countries (because it will have direct and indirect impacts on their economies), the rich countries can regain their normal rhythm within a short period, but developing countries will become poor and poorer.

Safe tourism

Airport and flight crew, transport from and to hotels, and hotel service crew with immune passports (cured Corona). Introduce special packages to travelers with immune passports. Promote the country as a corona safe destination.

Quarantine tourism

With the new evidence on COVID-19, scientists have a remote chance of inventing a vaccine and mitigating drugs in the coming several years. Hence, elders and patients with complicated diseases have to live with a high risk of infection and death. Offering exclusive packages for such people to spend holidays or vulnerable days in a safe touristic heaven may be a good attractive package for them.

We suggest a mix of open and close economy policy. We remain open to the best economic policies to adopt.

Inefficiency and corruption are observed in private and public sectors, though both are much higher in the government sector. Learned lessons are more than enough to form a policy-based action plan to bring about positive results.

Health net

All the students of medical and health sciences, current health professionals, and similar retired persons are automatically registered with the disaster management health task force. At the moment, there are about 8,000 health care students, 60,000 health care professionals, and 15,000 retired healthcare officers (Swiss Info May 10, 2020). On averagely, there is one healthcare worker for

70 families who can act as a health communicator and health educator in a disaster situation.

Every country should build an all-time (ever-ready) emergency task force (ETF). It is, too, a big lesson taught by the COVID-19 pandemic. Beginning of both semesters, the 1st of January and June, 20% of all health care institutes of the country should nominate 20% of their cadre to the ETF. Every worker should get an equal chance to join. No one is excused, even on medical grounds.

All non-medical employments should nominate 20% of their cadre for first aid and basic health education-three weeks course every year. The Ministry of Health should facilitate and coordinate the program. Government and private medical manufacturers, suppliers, distributors, whole-sellers, and retailers will be gazetted as all-time essential services and should provide facilities for smooth drug supply.

Three forces and police

first aid and basic health care education for all three forces and police should be made mandatory. Special training for establishing temporary hospitals, facilities and making the relevant equipment should be provided. Infrastructural material needed to build temporary healthcare facilities/hospitals should be made readily available. We can sell this service to the rest of the world when Sri Lanka has not an excess or as a humanitarian service. Since Sri Lanka is an island, Floating Hospitals can be built to render the service by moving faster and easier on sea routes to the disaster area, e.g. when heavy rains, floods, and landslides cause land blocks, a floating hospital anchored in Trincomalee can move to Galle easily and faster than getting aid through land routes or by air. Such medical services can be sold to Africa or any other country as a complete package in emergency situations (Staff + Facility). The patient could be brought to the ship by helicopter or by boat.

Nation Guard Force

A special task force (NGF) bearing no arms will be set up for humanitarian work during the disaster period. A special bill should be passed in parliament to allow chosen units of three forces to release their soldiers to the "Nation Guard Force" during the disaster period to engage in humanitarian work only. (If Sri Lanka had such a law during the time of civil war, the country would not have to face allegations of war crimes later. Retired police and military officers may be allowed to join the National Guard Force.)

Reproductive health should be properly addressed. An estimated 1,000 illegal abortions happen in a day. If the country is locked down for two months, the number of extra persons added to the population could be 60,000. Also, it should not be forgotten that long stays at home lead to more frequent sex engagements, which may increase pregnancies.

Sexual requirements of lonely people, those dissatisfied with usual engagements, and stress related to sex should be properly addressed. The free distribution or free availability of contraceptive methods is essential during a disaster period.

Hospitals will be subjected to special regulations under the Act. Every hospital must have a plan and preparedness to cater to a sudden regional disaster.

It is understood that some health and other professionals refrain from their duties to mitigate the disaster to avoid risk and hazards (to themselves). Special regulations to avoid such omissions and a system of imposing fines on such persons are required.

A special hotline and online windows for help in cases of domestic violence and burglary complaints and for counseling should be established.

Issue of substance addiction

Sri Lanka was estimated to have 120,000 heroin addicts and 700,000 cannabis addicts in 2019 (www.motortrafic.gov.lk, Total vehicle population 2007–2015). In all developing countries, they are a marginalized group of people with a high percentage of unemployment or living on daily wages, who engage in anti-social behavior like stealing, illegal deals, and underworld gangster activities. Surprisingly, in none of the countries, in which drug abuse is a major burden, has remarkable unrest been reported due to less availability (of drugs) and restricted movement that necessitated a special program for them.

Around the world, we have observed that there is a natural demand from people for social drinks, party drinks, recreational drinks, and something for bewildering (some extremists), etc.

I sense that this is a time to introduce a Recreational drinking culture. Instead of hard liquor and illegal "kasippu" (locally produced illegal arrack), wine and beer could be made available. Sometimes, this may be helpful in preventing youth from being attracted to hard drugs like heroin and cocaine.

Services to support children who witness abuse at home, and a domestic violence support service, awareness programs, and to attend to domestic accidents during a disaster are needed.

The essential drug reservoir should be maintained with the collaboration of the private sector. **A Pharmacy net** encompassing delivery and the dispensing system should be established. Online ordering and delivery systems should be planned with the support of the state and franchise pharmacy network.

Essential drugs should be produced in the country.

Transport net

Railway stations could act as (or be converted to) warehouses, wholesale, and transit centers for food. Special transport arrangements during the disaster period should be planned. Bus fares will be treble during the period to prevent unwanted movements by the passengers. Extra payments will be reimbursed by the workplace later. This will help to maintain social distancing. Allowance for bicycle and motorbike riders should be arranged.

According to the 2015 statistics, there are 2.9 million motorbikes and 5 million bicycles are in the country. Estimated figures for 2020 are 4.2 million motorbikes and 6 million bicycles and 1.4 million three-wheelers and 0.85 million motor cars (www.statistics.gov.lk, Economic statistics of Sri Lanka, 2016). Therefore, we can plan to more than 60% of the population to avoid public transport unnecessarily. All vehicles could transport more than five passengers, each automatically registered with the disaster management transport net – vehicle pool as they are first registered at Registrar of Motor Vehicles.

We recommend the government pay an allowance of Rs. 5,000 per month, all-time to echo-friendly riders (exclusive bicycle riders), Rs. 2,000 to motorbike riders, and Rs. 3,000 to electric three-wheelers and electric cars.

Different bus fares, high prices should be imposed during traffic hours. Traffic charges should be levied from luxury vehicles carrying less than two passengers. The app will be introduced to pay and monitor such movements.

There should be tax concessions for vehicles that carry over nine passengers and transportation of fewer than four people should be prohibited in them. In a disaster, all vehicles with more than seven seats in the region regulate under the operation center (with passes).

No free parking. We should encourage the use of bicycles and motor-bikes, which may benefit the riders in many ways, especially economically and health-wise.

Food net

Food security is one of the biggest requirements during any kind of disaster. A continuous supply of food to the affected area for all people in the community must be assured. In our proposal, we suggested an expert committee calculating per person consumption of essential foods and goods. For example, one person/week, 1.5 kg rice, 200 g sugar, etc., and then the provisions needed for a family per week. Fair and equitable food distribution should be maintained (again, the concept of communism will be implemented).

For that, supermarket networks will be expanded to very remote areas too. A special loan scheme to build infrastructure facilities in remote areas. Isolated retail shops will be networked. The retailers who have not obtained permits will be temporarily closed during the disaster period. Supermarket networks and networked retail shop networks will be aligned.

Prices of all the goods will be 10% less in areas below the poverty line and 10% higher in rich areas and neutral prices in middle-class zones. This will ensure the customers do not congregate in densely populated areas for buying foods and cash flow is ensured to rural areas. While supplying foods with no breach, we focus on the most essential foods. Grains (rice, green gram, mung, kaupi, etc.), yams (potatoes, manioc, sweet potatoes), sugar, and wheat flour. Mandatory reservoirs for six months should be maintained by the main producers, importers by law: Fruits (mango, banana), vegetables (jackfruit, breadfruit, others), and seed distribution for home gardening.

Identify the regions (soil, water, weather conditions, and skilled labor) suitable for the cultivation of essential crops and stay prepared to cultivate the required amount for the season. Under normal conditions, the essential crops which are not beneficial economically should not be cultivated. But model farms will be maintained. From them, high-quality value-added products will be produced in normal times while maintaining farming skills, agrotechnology, and nurseries for mass production.

A special loan and subsidy scheme should be established for the model farmers and importers of essential goods to maintain mandatory reservoirs. We suggest establishing non-governmental cooperation for paddy farmers and rice mills owners, vegetable farmers, and fruit farmers should network for organized cultivation, storing, transportation, and marketing of their goods.

Oil

Maintaining six months reserve is very essential for any country and storage facilities should be allocated. Sri Lanka has a great advantage of having an abundant oil storage facility in Trincomalee, which can be used after a little repair.

Administrative network

An efficient flow of executive orders from state leaders to the ground-level implementers is highly important in disaster management. A fully empowered combined operation Center for disaster management should be established.

Government sector employees of the affected area or country become the comrades of the special task force for disaster management. Sri Lanka has 2 million government servants (with three forces) to serve 5.6 million family units (www.statistics.gov.lk, Demographic and health survey report 2016). For efficient communication and coordination, one officer has to take care of only three families. This is a great advantage for the smooth flow of information, well-coordinated disaster mitigating work, and responsive network.

The operation center should coordinate all the networks of all possible stakeholders in the government, private, and NGO sectors. Among the duties of the operation center, we identify four major tusks

1 Demarcate the affected region (geographical boundary)
2 Identify the affected population
3 Identify the affected services
4 Identify and announce the tentative period

Education net

In Sri Lanka, there is a mixed system of government-controlled free education and a non-regulated private education system. Both are disorganized and not updated to global standards. There is still no widely accepted national policy on education too.

Online education is new to Sri Lanka but some experience in the field can count for the rapid implementation of a novel action plan. Though there is no census on digital literacy and the acquired digital facilities of the student population of the island, it is widely accepted that a significant percentage of both have significant deficiencies. However, it is not a reason for not starting and dispensing online education in the country in light of the pandemic. There are out-of-the-frame proposals to bring online education to all corners of the country such as laptops from mobile companies and financial institutes provided on competitive, easy payment methods and loan schemes, "pay after receiving a job in the future," etc. The government should be urged to provide such facilities nationwide.

All the teachers are requested to upload YouTube education materials according to the subjects they teach in school (40 minutes lessons for each topic). All students who have passed their advanced level, university teachers, and undergraduates, tuition masters could be requested to upload creative subject relevant lessons. This will bring them an additional income too.

Information net

Apex Information Center should be established with immediate effect in any disaster. Data collecting, analyzing, researching, and disseminating are the major duties of the center. Disaster management media ethics will be introduced to traditional media and social media. A special volunteer regulatory group will be set up among social media activists to monitor and regulate the circulation of wrong and harmful information. A similar regulatory body for digital and printed media was selected by themselves.

Media should broadcast model shows, advertisements, and programs briefing instructions on people's behavior, rules and regulations, and advantages and disadvantages of a disaster (not only talk shows). Independent polling, self-regulatory bodies for social and main media will be introduced. A religious council for religious and spiritual matters arising during the disaster will be introduced. It will be the focal point for policy recommendations to the government on related matters. It should be multi-religious proportionate to the population percentages.

Industrial net

Industries will be subjected to a special law in a disaster period. They should introduce a similar act as in the United States, which gives powers to order government and private industries to manufacture timely important products for disaster management during the said period only. A special low-interest loan scheme should be introduced to facilitate manufactures to manufacture substitutes as imports are restricted due to a disaster.

Bank of apparels

A special financial institute will be set up to look after the financial issues of the apparel industry. It would be a listed bank on Colombo Stock Exchange. Large, medium, small, micro (all types of) enterprises, all shareholders and owners, all executives of the industry should obtain shares in the bank.

This model could be used to safeguard and develop other industries with common interests. If the government has no proper plan for the national airline, this is the best time to resolve it. We can apply the same or suitable application to other loss-making government enterprises during a crisis period without much resistance from employees with a view to stopping further losses to the country. Every industry should obtain permits to keep their workplaces open by submitting a rational paper.

Conclusion

Successful management and mitigating of a pandemic or any kind of disaster mostly depend on early preparedness. A comprehensive disaster management plan backed by strong statutory powers is mandatory. Providing the basic daily needs of people without interruption is the focus. For that, we propose eight networked bodies, namely finance, food, health, transport, education, administration, industrial, and information nets to cover them. The whole community working as one to overcome the challenges during a disaster is highly essential. The pandemic is an opportunity that should not be missed by the developing countries looking to rise to the club of rich countries.

References

K. McCain, 2015, Nothing as Practical as a Good Theory, Does Lewis Maxim Still Have Salience in the Applied Social Science. Proceedings of the Association for Information Science and Technology. Volume 5, issue I, pages 1–4. https://doi.org/10.1002/pra2.2015.145052010077

B. Senanayaka, T. Darshana, Handbook of drug abuse information, 2019, National Dangerous Drugs Control Board, Sri Lanka.

Swiss Info, Online newspaper, Switzerland, May 10, 2020.

www.statistics.gov.lk, Demographic and health survey report 2016.

www.statistics.gov.lk, Economic statistics of Sri Lanka, 2016, page 5.

www.motortrafic.gov.lk, Total vehicle population 2007–2015.

6 COVID-19

An enabler for digital acceleration

Rasitha Wickramasinghe

Introduction

COVID-19 has been a change agent of global scale. It is an unprecedented event that forced the global economy to shut down for several months with families confined to their homes. Driven by these unique circumstances, individuals, communities, businesses, and governments found new ways to go about their daily activities. A majority of these changes were enabled by digital technology because of the physical distancing forced on us by the COVID-19 virus. In this chapter, we explore the role played by digital technology in facilitating some of the behavioral changes, and how COVID-19 can become an accelerator for digital adoption.

What is digital?

What comes to your mind when you hear the word "digital?" I tested it out on my family and here are the results: my 10-year-old son said "digital is a clock," his 13-year-old brother said "digital means ICT (information communication technology)" and my wife's answer was "digital is electronics and automation." They were all keen to know who was right. The truth is digital encompasses all the above, and more!

At the heart of digital is the theory of Boolean algebra, where information is represented by a series of signals expressed by "1"s and "0"s. Early adoption of Boolean logic for computing used vacuum tubes that took up large spaces but had limited processing power. However, the invention of the transistor and integrated circuits or ICs (that could pack thousands of transistors into a tiny space) increased the processing power by several magnitudes and heralded the transition from an analog world to a digital world. Since the 1970s, electronic clocks, watches, dictionaries, radios, home appliances to medical equipment have been replacing their analog counterparts, and digital technology has become an omnipresent part of human life.

A brief history of digital

The world's first general-purpose computer, ENIAC invented in 1945, consisted of 18,000 vacuum tubes. It was purposely built to calculate the trajectory of artillery during Second World War and could perform what humans would take

DOI: 10.4324/9781003197416-6

a day to perform within thirty minutes. Although impressive for its time, the main drawbacks of vacuum tube computing were large space requirements relative to processing power, high energy consumption, and limited reliability. The ENIAC, for example, despite taking an entire room and weighing 30 tons, was equivalent to a modern-day "Angry Bird" application in terms of its processing power [1].

Transistor and electronic chips

A pivotal moment in our digital journey was the invention of the transistor at Bell Labs in 1947 by William Shockley, John Bardeen, and Walter Brattain. Transistors have become the fundamental building block of modern-day computing along with IC technology that allows millions of transistors to be packed into a small silicon wafer. The more transistors there are in a chip, the greater the processing power.

The original transistor built in 1947 was large enough that it was pieced together by hand. By contrast, more than 6 million transistors (of 22 nm technology) could fit in the period at the end of this sentence [1]. This trend of increasing computing power and decreasing relative costs was first observed by Intel founder Gordon Moore. In 1965, he predicted the number of transistors in an electronic chip would double every two years and as result, the processing power would increase at an exponential pace, while relative costs would decrease [2]. Commonly referred to as Moore's Law, this became the golden rule for the electronics industry, and a springboard for innovation.

As an example, compared to Intel's first microprocessor, the 4004 introduced in 1971, a 14 nm microprocessor available today provides 3,500 times more performance, is 90,000 times more energy efficient, and price per transistor has fallen more than 60,000 times [2]. The A13 chip that powers iPhone 11 today has a staggering 8.5 billion transistors [3]. If the car industry had evolved at the same rate as the electronics industry, today cars would travel at a speed of 480,000 km per hour, and have a fuel efficiency of more than 840,000 km per liter, and would cost less than 4 cents [2].

Personal computer and network era

Moore's Law predicted the computer processing power could be infinite, and therefore the limiting factor in harnessing this power was software. In the early 1970s, during an era of mainframes (computers that took up several thousand square feet), asked the question, "What if there is a computer in every household?" With that began the personal computer (PC) revolution and Windows operating system developed by Gates's Microsoft Corporation that has dominated the PC market for nearly four decades. According to Statista, the installed base of PCs worldwide was approximately 1.5 billion in 2015 [4].

The next phase of digital evolution was inter-connected PCs or computer networks that allowed sharing of information and collaboration. Computer networks were first created for applications in the defense industry, universities, and businesses. A defining moment in the evolution of the network era was the invention of the Internet by British computer scientist Sir Tim Berners-Lee. Websites, web browsers, search engines, and acronyms such as HTTP (HyperText Transfer Protocol), URL (Universal Resource Locator), HTML (HyperText Marked-up Language) were all born out of what Sir Berners-Lee called the World Wide Web in 1990.

Three decades later, there are more than 1.8 billion websites and more than 4.5 billion people or nearly 60% of the world population is connected to the internet [5]. According to Indian government data, there are more than half a billion people connected to the internet in the last decade alone, and India now has twice as many internet users as the entire population of the United States. The internet has also turned our society into homebodies, individuals who do everything from the comfort of their homes (shopping, banking, learning, entertainment, information gathering, and much more) instead of venturing outdoors to complete tasks.

An added dimension to this connected world has been the introduction of mobile phones. Starting with GSM (Global System for Mobile) technology in the early 1990s, mobile phones have enabled anytime, anywhere connectivity for billions of people worldwide. The smartphone revolution started by Apple in 2007 and the continuous evolution of mobile technology from GSM to 3G (3rd generation) to 5G (5th generation) has revolutionized how humans communicate today. Traditional voice communication is now complemented or replaced by messaging and social network applications enabled by data networks.

Digital adoption

What drives people to adopt digital technology? Some of the primary drivers are that it helps to solve common consumer pain points and offers a better and faster experience. A digital radio may be preferred over an analog radio due to its smaller size, greater reliability, and ability to store channels, etc. Digital CDs offered better sound quality over radio cassettes, while digital music players such as iPods allowed the convenience of storing hundreds of songs into a device that would fit into a pocket. A smartphone is more portable and affordable than a PC and therefore is a preferred way of connecting to the world. The miniaturization, increased reliability, affordability, and accessibility are at the heart of the ubiquitous digital adoption we see today.

Digital natives and digital immigrants

Modern-day digital adoption by individuals can be broadly categorized into digital natives and digital immigrants. Digital Natives belonging to Millennial and Gen Z generations were born into the digital age. The internet is their natural habitat, performing all their social interactions, searching for information, making purchases, and even doing their homework online. Instant response, openness, and adaptability are their default digital standards [6].

In contrast, digital immigrants are late adopters of technology. Most were born before digital technology became pervasive and have adopted it to varying degrees later in their lives. They have come to accept the realities of the digital revolution and are willing to understand its role in modern life and learn. For example, my wife's parents born in the 1950s, have increased their digital adoption as technology became simpler and more intuitive. Today they are proficient digital immigrants connecting with their global circle of friends and family via WhatsApp, Zoom, and other social network applications. In contrast, my mother born in the 1930s is a digital alien that has never ventured into the world of technology, preferring traditional wall clock, transistor radio, newspaper, and fixed-line telephony, over their digital counterparts.

A great example of a digital immigrant I met recently was Jorge, an Uber driver in Colombo. He is 60 years old, had worked at the Grand Hotel, Nuwaraeliya, a leading hotel with a rich heritage in the central region of Sri Lanka, for over 25 years. He used a feature phone for voice but had never used a smartphone in his life until last year. He spent 15,000 Sri Lankan Rupees to buy a smartphone so that he could register as an Uber driver to top up his pension. He currently works 5.5 days per week and earns approximately 90,000 Sri Lankan Rupees per month to supplement his retirement income.

Visionaries to laggards

Organizations can also be categorized by the extent of their technology adoption, just as individuals. One of the most celebrated works in this field was carried out by American thought leader Geoffrey Moore [6]. He classifies five types of leaders by technology adoption.

- Visionaries – excited by the possibilities of technology advancement and looks five to ten years into the future.
- Early adopters – convinced by future vision articulated by visionaries, look to embrace technology to create new products/services or generate greater operating efficiency.
- Early majority – the trend spotters that see early traction in a technology and is quick to embrace to create a competitive advantage for the organization.
- Late majority – risk averse and wait for technology to be mainstream before considering adoption.
- Laggards – not convinced by benefits of technology or have vested interests and therefore provide reasons and excuses why technology should not be adopted.

In his 1980s best-selling book *Crossing the Chasm*, Geoffrey Moore [7] argues the greatest challenge facing technology companies is getting a critical mass of customers for its products or services from early adopters to early majority, the so-called crossing of the chasm [8].

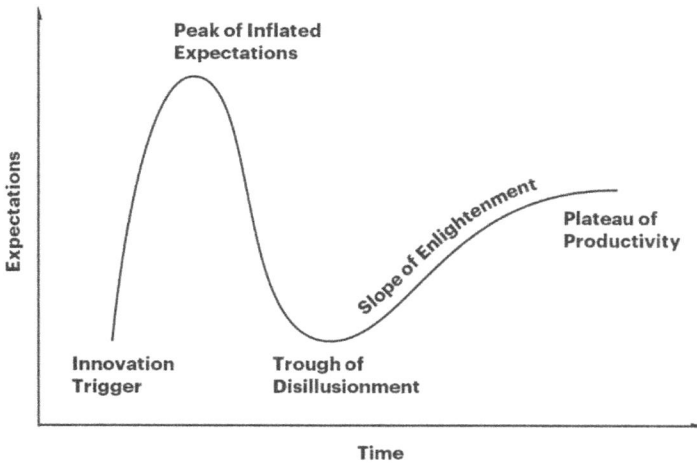

Figure 6.1 Gartner's Hype Cycle.

Source: Gartner, https://www.gartner.com/en/research/methodologies/gartner-hype-cycle

Bill Gates (Gates, 2018) summed up technology adoption when he stated, "Most people overestimate what they can do in one year and underestimate what they can do in ten years." Gartner's "Hype Cycle" [9] reinforces this thesis, where a majority of technologies early on fail to live up to the peak of inflated expectations, resulting in a trough of disillusionment, eventually maturing to deliver expected benefits at affordable costs over the longer run as presented in Figure 6.1.

Digitally enabled world: Pre-COVID

During the last three decades, unprecedented digital adoption has taken place in spite of pandemics (SARS and MERS outbreaks), economic crisis (crash of the dot com bubble in 2000 and global financial crisis in 2008), and continued geo-political instabilities (9/11 terror attacks, Iraq War, Brexit, US-China trade war, etc.).

SCAM (Social, Cloud, Analytics, and Mobile)

At the heart of this digital adoption is mobile technology. According to GSMA, there are over 5 billion unique mobile subscribers globally, out of which 60% are smartphone users. There are over 3.6 billion mobile internet users today and that will grow to 5 billion users by 2025. This provides unprecedented access to a global user base, helping to generate exponential growth for technology applications and platforms. There are more than 9 billion "internet-of-things" (IoT) devices connecting homes, factories, and cities to the internet. This is projected to grow to a staggering 25 billion devices by 2025.

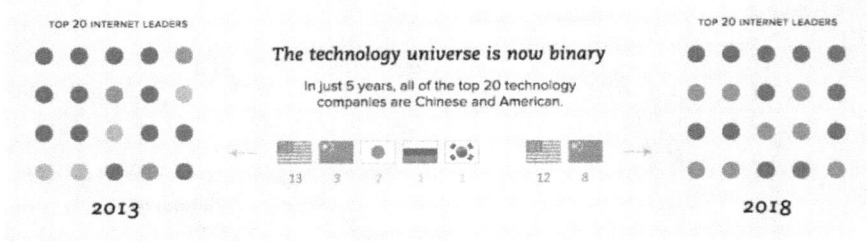

Figure 6.2 Top 20 Technology Companies.

Source: Mary Meeker's famous Internet Trends 2018, Kleiner Perkins, https://www.kleinerperkins.com/perspectives/internet-trends-report-2018/

SCAM or Social, Cloud, Analytics, and Mobile have in fact been the big digital trends over the last decade. For example, businesses spent nearly $230 billion globally in 2019 on the cloud, according to Gartner, and this could increase to as much as $355 billion by 2022. These trends have enabled technology giants to emerge from the two largest economies of the world but serving global audiences: the FAANG (Facebook, Apple, Amazon, Netflix, and Google) in the United States and BAT (Baidu, Alibaba, and Tencent) in China. As per Mary Meeker's famous Internet Trends 2018 report [10], the top 20 largest tech giants by valuation now hail entirely from the United States and China (Figure 6.2) [11].

Other nascent technologies

In addition to SCAM, multiple other technologies have come to the forefront over the recent years. These include technologies such as artificial intelligence (AI), Robotics, IoT that enable smart homes, factories and cities, autonomous vehicles, drones, 3D printing blockchain, and quantum computing, just to name a few.

Acquisitions made by tech giants are a good indication of the next wave of emerging technologies. For example, since 2010, 6 US tech giants have made a total of 66 acquisitions in the AI space (Apple 20, Google 14, Microsoft 10, Intel 9, Facebook 8, and Amazon 5). In May 2020, Apple confirmed it acquired NextVR, a startup that provides sports and other content for virtual-reality headsets [12]. In Jan 2020, Visa announced that it is buying fintech startup Plaid that connects various payment apps signaling Visa's continued push into the fintech space.

Vision unveiled by incumbent tech giants also indicates the direction in which technology is moving. For example, Google CEO Sundar Pichai stated in May 2019, "We are moving from a company that helps you find answers to a company that helps you get things done." In January 2020, Amazon's founder Jeff Bezos claimed, "Today, online commerce saves customers money and precious time. Tomorrow, through personalization, online commerce will accelerate the very process of discovery." Both these statements point toward a world where AI will play a bigger role in the future [13].

Human behavior and social norms

Today's human population is made up of multiple generations with varying degrees of digital exposure and adaptability as discussed earlier. From digital immigrants to digital natives and visionaries to laggards, how humans embrace technology differs based on familiarity, level of comfort, access, and necessity [7]. While my 82-year-old mother has never operated a computer or mobile phone in her life, my 13-year-old son can teach me the most obscure features on my smartphone and introduce me to educational YouTube channels such as Vox and TedEd.

A social norm adopted during the last century is the five-day workweek. First introduced by industrialist Henry Ford, the five-day workweek was enshrined into American law in 1940. Gradually other nations followed, although some countries such as China only started recognizing the five-day workweek as recently as 1995 [14]. Commuting to work and surviving Monday–Friday had become a norm for the global workforce.

The Monday–Friday routine (with truncated hours) had also become the norm for primary, secondary, and tertiary education, where a lion's share of learning was confined to the classrooms. Despite significant improvements in digital connectivity and related applications over the last decade, the majority of global households had resigned themselves to the five-day, 9 am–5 pm work/school routine. Sacrificing 20%–30% of productive time on a daily commute (assuming eight hours of sleep and one to three hours of commuting per day) was considered a necessity and a social norm. Weekend was the oasis that every family escaped to recover and recharge to repeat the same cycle all over again the following week.

Over the last two decades, e-commerce has emerged as an alternative consumer channel. Despite the rapid rise of e-commerce, the preferred mode of shopping for greater majority of consumers remains brick and mortar stores. Similarly, banks have introduced multiple digital channels, but there are generations of customers that still feel the need to visit a branch to do banking. Weekend trips to grocery stores, shopping malls, or watching a movie in cinema were also social norms for the modern consumers, despite the availability of online options [15]. Cash was a necessity despite multiple digital payments available and healthcare was only effective if patients could be physically examined. Even personal training or personal tutoring had to be conducted one-to-one with physical presence, and doing these activities remotely was inconceivable.

While digital has become an omnipresent part of our daily lives, not even the most optimistic digital visionary would have thought of giving up the physical world to a virtual world, seven days a week. The "herd mentality" forced us to conform to tradition despite there being plenty of evidence to suggest that there may be more productive and environmentally friendly ways to go about our daily lives. The global wisdom was the majority of human activity must take place in the real world with physical presence, with digitally enabled virtual world complementing for occasional convenience. This notion was challenged by the pandemic for multiple generations and nations across the globe.

Post-COVID digital acceleration

As we know it now, COVID-19 has been a change agent of global scale. Microsoft CEO Satya Nadella summed it up well during his quarterly earnings report to Wall Street in April 2020, when he called out, "We've seen two years' worth of digital transformation in two months" [16]. In fact, this statement epitomizes digital acceleration: a digital transformation that would have taken several years, takes place over a much shorter duration driven by necessity.

As a result of the pandemic, multiple institutions were digitally transformed during lockdown. Companies, government organizations, schools, and universities were all forced to function remotely. Shopping, entertainment, fitness, banking to dining had to rely on online platforms to keep their businesses functioning [17]. In a post-pandemic era, as the world moves to a "remote everything" model [18], we explore how some key areas such as work, education, shopping, entertainment, and healthcare are being digitally accelerated.

Workplace

After sleep, work is where we spend majority of our lifetime. Assuming an average person lives up to approximately 80 years, 13.5 years of our life is spent at work (compared to 33.5 years we spend sleeping) [15]. Not only does work provide us with financial security, but it also creates a social network outside of our immediate family and friends. This is proven by multiple social surveys since 1973 that have consistently shown at least two-thirds of individuals will continue to work even if they were to win $10 million lottery, demonstrating motivation for work stretches far beyond financial security [19].

Automation

Even prior to COVID-19 outbreak, there was increased scrutiny of jobs and the workplace due to emerging technology trends such as AI, robotics and 3D printing. For example, OECD predicted nearly 14% of jobs in OECD countries are likely to be automated, while another 32% are at high risk of being partially automated – so nearly one in two people are likely to be affected in some way [19]. Expressing his views on the future of work with Wharton University in July 2019, Ravi Kumar, President of Infosys, stated, "Two big shifts on the jobs front: repetitive tasks to non-repetitive tasks, and from problem-solving to problem-finding. We have to move to a continuum of lifelong learning" [20].

An example of such workplace automation was Telefónica Perú that automated more than 6 million high-friction and low-value calls every month by using intelligent digital agents to man customer service lines and carry out tasks, such as helping users activate their SIM cards. This freed up human customer service reps to focus on value adding tasks, thus allowing departmental goals to be met and maintain a positive impact for employees [16]. A similar example of using digital assistant to automate repetitive tasks was the service desk at US information technology company Unisys with more than 150,000 callers per month. By using a digital employee that can speak in both voice and text, Unisys was able to deflect 32% of the calls from the service desk, allowing the human service desk team to focus on solving problems that are a bit more complex than a password reset [21].

Remote working

It was estimated that 2.7 billion people or more than four out of five in the global workforce were affected by lockdowns restricting travel to the workplace [22]. As pointed out earlier, majority of employees spend 20%–30% of productive time commuting, therefore just avoiding commutes alone reduces stress and gives employees more time.

In a 2018 survey, 76% of public and private sector employees indicated they would be more loyal to their employers if they had flexible work options. In fact, a survey of US internet users carried out as far back as 2014, two-thirds of respondents indicated that they are actually more productive when they work remotely [23]. The Office of Personnel Management's 2018 Report on the status of telework in the US federal government found that 63% of respondents believed telework improved their performance [24].

The following graphic is a good illustration of how the future of work is evolving in Figure 6.3: The myth that employees need to be in an office environment, working 9 am–5 pm, five days of the week to be productive was firmly challenged with countries going into lockdown. Overnight workforces were adapting to remote work using various communication applications and platforms. In my organization, a global management consultancy with more than 150 employees across offices in the United States and Sri Lanka, the shift to 100% remote working happened over a weekend with hardly a glitch. Following this transition, most employees were putting in 10–12 hour workdays, unable to define boundaries of personal life and work life given that both were now functioning from the same place, the home.

Gartner's analysis shows that 48% of employees will likely work remotely at least part of the time after the COVID-19 pandemic, compared to 30% pre-pandemic. In fact, 74% of CFOs intend to increase remote work at their organization after the outbreak [25], and large tech companies are taking the lead in this regard. Twitter CEO Jack Dorsey acknowledged that when the company reopens its offices, it will not be an immediate return to normal and is allowing employees to work from home indefinitely. Facebook will reportedly limit its office capacity to 25% of the workforce when it reopens offices, with cafeteria

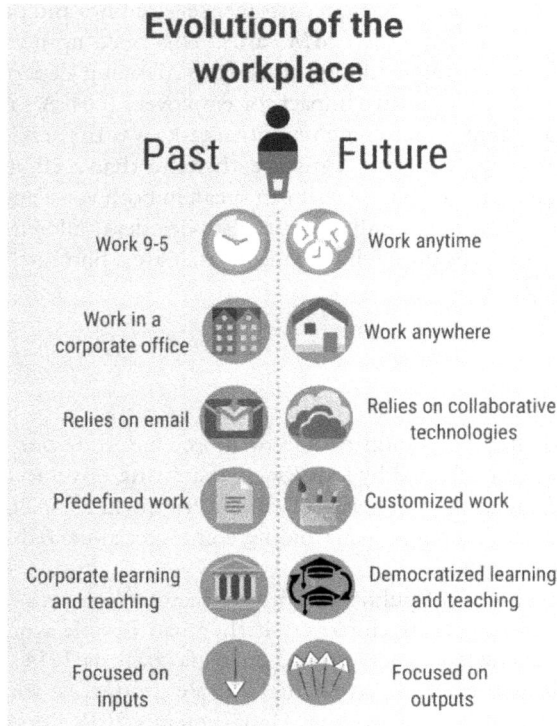

Evolution of the workplace

Past   Future

Past			Future
Work 9-5			Work anytime
Work in a corporate office			Work anywhere
Relies on email			Relies on collaborative technologies
Predefined work			Customized work
Corporate learning and teaching			Democratized learning and teaching
Focused on inputs			Focused on outputs

Figure 6.3 Diagram on the Evolution of the Workplace Patterns.

Source: Adapted from *The Future of Work: Attract New Talent, Build Better Leaders, and Create a Competitive Organization*, by Jacob Morgan, Wiley; 1st Edition (August 25, 2014).

meals replaced by grab-and-go meals and outside visitors banned from entry at the outset.

So, by all accounts, remote working is here to stay and organizations that recognize this shift are likely to benefit over organizations that go back to 100% office-based "old normal." Mahesh Amalean, a visionary business leader and co-founder of MAS Holdings, one of South Asia's leading apparel manufacturers headquartered in Sri Lanka, echoed this view in a Twitter message shown in Figure 6.4.

In remote-enabled future organizations, a key differentiator will be organization culture. Organizations that have a self-motivated workforce driven by a transformational purpose will create "high-trust networks" that are highly productive and efficient while optimizing operational overheads. In contrast, traditional organizations will go back to the pre-COVID normal of high operation overheads and "low-trust networks" that rely on command-control culture to get things done.

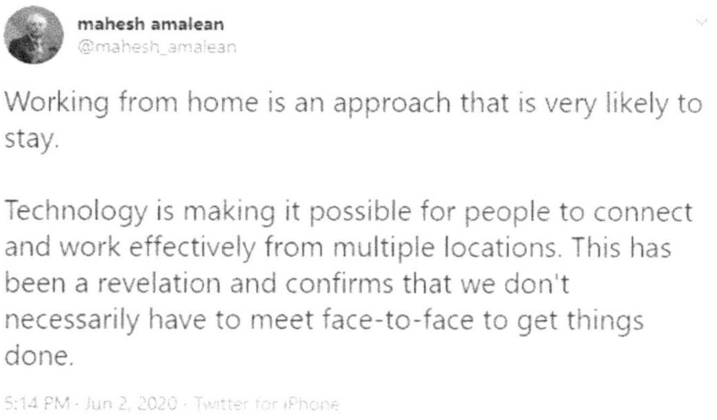

mahesh amalean
@mahesh_amalean

Working from home is an approach that is very likely to stay.

Technology is making it possible for people to connect and work effectively from multiple locations. This has been a revelation and confirms that we don't necessarily have to meet face-to-face to get things done.

5:14 PM · Jun 2, 2020 · Twitter for iPhone

Figure 6.4 Coronavirus Makes Work From Home (WFH) the New Normal.

Source: Twitter, https://twitter.com/mahesh_amalean/status/1267784039689265153

Virtual meetings

Physical meeting rooms were one facility that all organizations could not have enough of. I can recall the number of times I have been forced to complete meetings in corridors or walk to the nearest coffee shop due to the lack of available meeting spaces. In a remote working environment, the frequency or the number of participants is no longer a constraint, as long as all participants have access to a decent internet connection.

Microsoft Teams and Zoom have become the ultimate winners of this virtual meeting revolution. Some of the numbers Satya Nadella shared during April's investor call were staggering: 200 million Microsoft Teams meeting participants in a single day, generating more than 4.1 billion meeting minutes. Microsoft Teams now has a 75 million active user base, amongst them 20 organizations with more than 100,000 users and 183,000 Educational organizations. You can video chat with up to 250 people at once with Microsoft Teams, or present live to up to 10,000 people [26]. On Zoom, up to 1,000 users can participate in a single video call, and 49 videos can appear on the screen at once. Annual user conferences and company annual general meetings (AGMs) with several thousand participants are shifting online due to social distancing protocols imposed in a post-pandemic era.

One important ingredient for a successful virtual meeting is video technology. As an example, the MD of my organization would insist that every participant enable video during virtual meetings and replace emails with Microsoft Teams messages for all internal communications.

According to Microsoft, the use of video for virtual meetings vary based on geography. The most active Microsoft Teams users were in Norway and the Netherlands with about 60% of calls conducted using video. Australians use video in meetings

57% of the time, Italy 53%, Chile 52%, Switzerland 51%, and Spain 49%. Meanwhile, people in the UK, Canada, and Sweden use video 47% of the time and people in Mexico and the United States use it 41% and 38%, respectively [27].

In contrast, India uses video in 22% of meetings, Singapore 26%, South Africa 36%, France 37%, and Japan 39%. This may be attributed in part to limited access to devices and stable internet connections in some regions such as India and South Africa. Other reasons may include lack of suitable workspaces at home, the power distance within an organization, and cultural norms.

As remote working and virtual meetings become the norm, hiring and firing are also shifting online. Even before the pandemic, my organization made use of video technology for recruitment by requesting candidates to submit a two-minute video to describe themselves and their interests. As nations went into lockdown, new employees joining organizations had to acquaint their new colleagues virtually. Ice breakers such as #guessthelocation by looking at travel photos, online treasure hunts, or conversation sparked by an object of mutual interest had become some of the ways of getting to know colleagues virtually, according to new article published by BBC in June 2020 [27]. Some of the businesses hardest hit by the pandemic such as ones in the travel industry had also resorted to "firing employees over Zoom" as the pandemic started to affect their businesses, far from an ideal situation [28].

Effects of remote working

As organizations embrace new modes of working, parts of the old ecosystems will get disturbed. Commercial real estate and business travel are perhaps two industries that will be the hardest hit. Due to the availability of superior teleconferencing facilities and cost rationalization, some of the domestic and international travel will never return. Former CEO of Spirit Airlines Ben Baldanza predicts that 5%–10% of business air travel will be lost permanently as a result of the pandemic.

Increased utilization of location-independent contractors or gig economy workers that provide employers with greater flexibility is another likely trend in post-COVID workplaces. A recent Gartner survey revealed that 32% of organizations are replacing full-time employees with contingent workers as a cost-saving measure [26]. Utilizing more gig workers provides employers with greater workforce management flexibility.

In the medium and longer term, these organizations will also realize that the functions they have made remote-capable can also be performed by highly skilled workers in lower-cost countries. In short, jobs will first move from in-person to remote-domestic, and eventually to remote-overseas.

Education

According how we spend our life study referred to earlier [15], an average person spends less than a year (334 days to be exact) on primary and secondary education. Despite this being significantly lower than the 13.5 years we spend at the workplace, it is still substantial given the time can be spread over 10–13 year period of our lives.

Albert Einstein, during his visit to Boston in 1921, while commenting on college education, stated, "Education is not the learning of facts, but the training of minds to think." The current education system was introduced more than 200 years ago to suit the needs of the industrial age and its relevance for modern day needs was under scrutiny long before the outbreak of COVID-19. For example, some critics have suggested current universities as the next site of reformation, citing parallels between dispensation of academic credentials to the dispensation of indulgences by Roman Catholic church in the 16th century. Harvard Business School professor Clayton Christensen, regarded as the pioneer of digital disruption theory, predicted in 2017 that "50 percent of the 4,000 colleges and universities in the U.S. will be bankrupt in 10 to 15 years."[29]

While there is a lot being debated about how the current education system needs to evolve to meet future demands of the world, for the purposes of this investigation, we focus on the iron triangle of education: quality, access, and cost and how the pandemic may accelerate some of the disruptive trends that were already in motion.

Quality of education

As referenced earlier, Infosys President Ravi Kumar predicts "a continuum of lifelong learning" or "perpetual student" as the future of education. When I reflect on this statement, it dawns on me that I have gained more knowledge in the last 5 years than during the previous 45 years of my life, primarily enabled by digital learning tools that are at my disposal.

A good example of how digital tools are aiding the quality of education is the self-guided, online social studies course "Big History Project" created by historian David Christian, which covers almost 14 billion years of history, starting with the big bang. Through a six-hour journey of text, audio, and video material covering eight threshold moments of history, Christian summarizes the origins of the universe to modern-day life that can be a substitute for several months of text-based classroom learning. Bill Gates calls it "my favorite course of all time," and his May 2018 blog post went on to say [30].

> Big History tells the story of the universe from the big bang to the first signs of life to today's complex societies. It shows how everything is connected to everything else, weaving together insights and evidence from across disciplines into a single, understandable narrative [8].

In an effort to individualize learning, China has launched one of the most ambitious classroom technology experiments the world has seen to date. Primary and secondary school students in a Shanghai-based school wear brain wave sensing headbands that measure student's attention and concentration at ten minute intervals. Classroom robots measure the health and engagements levels of students, chip-enabled uniforms track the location of students, and surveillance cameras monitor students' behavior. A combination of IoT, analytics, and AI collects multiple data points that provide teachers information on areas students need help to create a differentiated and personalized learning experience [31].

Technologies such as Virtual Reality headsets are providing students immersive learning experiences that increase the speed and effectiveness of learning. Online assessments and automation of administrative tasks are also allowing teachers more time to develop better relationships with students improving the quality of education delivered.

Access to education

Although technology had been introduced into the classrooms over the years, education was pigeonholed as a discipline that needed physical interaction. Unlike workplace where employers and employees had experimented with various degrees of remote working, education was largely delivered in the physical realms of a classroom. At the peak of lockdown in mid-April, 90% of enrolled learners or 1.6 billion students across 194 countries were affected by the pandemic [32]. The pandemic has done more to make distance learning a reality in a few short months than the combined efforts of the previous decade, when remote learning was a "nice-to-have" rather than a "need-to-have."

Overnight schools have equipped teachers and learners with connected technology, mobile and internet service providers have increased their reach and capacity, even lowering prices to increase affordability, while some content providers have offered free access to educational material. The Indian online learning app Byju's has a user base of more than 50 million using its products, which range from interactive video lessons, live classes, quizzes, and exam preparation. Nearly 25% of Byju's users had joined in March and April 2020 when free access was provided to the platform [33].

Overall, understandings about the need for connectivity and the technical and human foundations that make distance learning possible have shifted considerably over the last six months and are quickly ushering in a new era for education. The ability of educators to provide access to distance learning is dependent on a multitude of factors that include:

- Access to national educational platforms delivered over broadcast and online platforms as well as limitations in household access to electricity, TV, radio, digital devices, and internet connectivity.
- Availability of learning materials aligned with national curricula that can be delivered through broadcast and online platforms.
- Preparedness of teachers to deliver such content over digital platforms and availability and ability of parents or guardians to facilitate effective home-based distance learning.
- Ability to monitor access to distance learning, track interruptions to learning, and evaluate learning outcomes.

Emerging anecdotal evidence suggests that, while delivering educational programs remotely ensures some degree of continuity of learning for many students, absenteeism of students from online learning or disengagement from courses despite logging-in are not uncommon. Even in a European country heavily affected by the COVID-19 pandemic with a better ICT readiness, the absenteeism rate from online learning has been between 5% and 10%.

As many as 465 million children and youth, or almost 47% of all primary and secondary students being targeted by national online learning platforms, do not have access to the internet at home. While the share of students with no access to internet at home is less than 15% in Western Europe and North America, it is as high as 80% in sub-Saharan Africa. It is also worth noting that the average share of households with computer access around the world is 53%, demonstrating the reliance on mobile devices for remote learning. However, some of the trends observed are encouraging. For example, when Byju's launched in India in 2015, only one in four Indians had access to the internet. Now it has increased to one in two, and 60% of Byju's users are from outside the ten largest cities in India, showcasing the power of technology to reduce the education gap.

The global e-learning industry is estimated to grow to more than $350 billion by 2025, 3.5× growth compared to $100 billion market in 2015. Worldwide Education app downloads increased 90% during peak week in March 2020, compared to a weekly average of Q4 2019.

Snapask is a Hong Kong-based e-learning platform that helps students to ask questions and get answers from more than 300,000 online tutors. It applies machine learning and mobile cloud services to make education more effective, with personalized content recommendations based on students' revision habits and learning progress. More than 30% of 3.5 million Snapask users joined during February/March 2020, and the average time they spend on the platform has also increased by 40% compared to the same time last year, according to Snapask CEO Timothy Yu [34].

Learn In is an upskilling-as-a-service platform helping organizations with their large-scale, internal upskilling initiatives by helping them manage the financing, time, program selection, and candidate selection considerations across the organization [35]. This US startup was launched right at the start of the pandemic; it is a proactive upskilling option for organizations to send employees for training at reduced or no pay and bring back to the workforce at a later date, rather than laying them off.

The University of Arizona Global Campus is an example of how access to university education is extended across the globe. The program was expanded when international travel restrictions and visa moratoriums were put in place due to COVID-19. The University of Arizona Global Campus is now available across 5 continents in 34 countries (including China, Ireland, Mexico, the United Arab Emirates, India, and Japan), offering 10 customized degree paths to more than 200 undergraduate majors, 10 graduate certificates, and 60 fully online degrees at both the undergraduate and graduate levels [36].

According to University of Arizona President Robert C. Robbins, "The Global Campus is a long-term effort towards meeting the United Nations' sustainable development goal of providing accessible quality education to the world. We are truly making affordable, world-class education available to global citizens around the world and, in this time of the COVID-19 pandemic, it has never been needed more." [10].

Such global initiatives can increase access to foreign tertiary students. The number of enrolled foreign tertiary students worldwide increased by nearly five-fold from 1980 to 2014. However, of the 5.3 million students studying outside their place of origin, 3.6 million come from OECD countries [37]. E-learning platforms such as University Arizona Global Campus can increase access to students in emerging markets.

Cost of education

The digitization of education and access to it is likely to accelerate in a post-COVID world. COVID-19 is likely to emerge as the threshold moment that showed the world education does not necessarily need to be confined to the realms of physical classrooms but a lot more can be done online.

Even prior to COVID-19, there were significant questions marks over university education. In the United States, for example, the average cost of a university degree had risen 2.5 times over the last decade and the average student debt for the class of 2018 was $29,200 [36]. The emergence of MOOC (massive open online courses) platforms such as Udemy, Coursera had already brought down the cost of education prior to the pandemic. As pandemic forced brick and mortar universities to go online, students and parents were starting to question their value over online MOOC platforms.

The worldwide remote learning experiment triggered by the pandemic may demonstrate that primary to tertiary education can function effectively using a blend of online and offline experiences, at a fraction of historical costs. If it does, it may lead to a reckoning that transforms the delivery of education, particularly for universities, as students begin to weigh the costs and benefits of a four-year residential experience to an online education that is of shorter duration that offer specific skills desired by potential future employers.

Google's announcement of 100,000 scholarships for online certificates in data analytics, project management, and UX in July 2020 is a great example of how quality, access, and cost of education is changing [38]. The courses are offered through the online learning platform Coursera, taught by Google employees, can be completed in three to six months and certificates will be considered as the equivalent of a four-year college degree for related roles at the company.

Other lifestyle aspects

Visits to physical stores and malls were a habit of global consumers in a pre-COVID world. The average time spent by Americans in a mall was 135 minutes, and 56% of adult Americans reported visiting a mall in the previous 30 days [39]. The time Europeans spend on shopping and personal services (like visiting a doctor or a hairdresser) ranged from 17 minutes per day in Romania to 35 minutes in Germany, according to a survey carried out in 15 EU countries between 2008 and 2015 [40].

In a post-COVID world, we can expect two major consumer shifts: consumer spending shifting to essential purchases as economic headwinds of the pandemic affect global consumers, secondly the acceleration of e-commerce driven by social restrictions and physical separation. Retailers with strong platforms and sophisticated data analysis are better placed in connecting with consumers and offering them value-added services in a post-COVID world. Trends such as unmanned retail stores for experiential purchases, buy-online-pickup-in-store (BOPIS), "dark stores" acting as mini-fulfillment centers may become the future of retail. Amazon and Alibaba have become big winners of e-commerce acceleration with Amazon's gross merchandize value (GMV) exceeding $1 trillion and Alibaba increasing its like for sales for the quarter ending in March 2020 by 22% [41].

Telemedicine is another area that is set to accelerate as a result of the pandemic. For example, the struggling Sri Lankan telemedicine app oDoc got a new lease of life in the immediate aftermath of COVID-19, registering hundreds of new doctors and patients to its platform and launching Sri Lanka National Telemedicine Service in March 2020, in association with Ministry of Health and GMOA (Government Medical Officers' Association) [42]. Doctors in the United States can now perform remote visits across state boundaries, video chat or email patients in compliance with HIPAA and healthcare insurance providers are now obliged to reimburse expenses for telemedicine services. Telehealth offerings are also expected to improve with at-home testing and diagnostics becoming more accessible and affordable and the proliferation of medical wearables for remote monitoring of patients and their symptoms.

Another trend we will witness in a post-COVID world is the advertising spend shifting from traditional broadcast media to online channels. According to GroupM, a subsidiary of global advertising firm WPP, for the first time, digital marketing is predicted to account for more than half the $530 billion global advertising industry in 2020 (excluding online ads sold by old media outlets such as news publishers or broadcasters). The shift toward online advertising acceleration during the pandemic is expected to be greater than the impact of television on the advertising industry during the 20th century. As advertisers seek less expensive alternatives, overall global spending is predicted to decline by nearly 12%, with spending on traditional channels declining by more than 20%. In comparison, digital marketing channels boosted by greater online activity is expected to decline by less than 3% during 2020 [43].

As digital activity increased due to COVID-19, it also became an opportunity for unscrupulous elements to spread misinformation and fraud. The World Health Information (WHO) warned that it has been fighting a war on two fronts – the actual pandemic, and an "infodemic" of myths, rumors, and "false prevention measures, or cures" being spread on social media. Global messaging platform WhatsApp limited the forwarding of messages to one contact at a time to curb the spread of misinformation. UK's National Cyber Security Centre (NCSC) announced in April 2020 that it had taken down more than 2,000 COVID-19 related scams in a single month. These scams included stores selling fraudulent coronavirus related items, websites trying to launch malware on visitors, phishing sites seeking personal information such as passwords or credit card details, and "advance-fee frauds" where victims are duped into handing over a "set-up" payment in the belief they'll get a large sum in return.

Conclusions

The COVID-19 pandemic is a threshold moment in human history. No event of such magnitude has been experienced by multiple generations born after the Second World War. The "physical distancing" of COVID-19 is forcing us to do things differently, thereby addressing one of the most challenging aspects of digital adoption: changing behaviors and social norms. In other words, COVID-19 has generated "two years' worth of digital transformations inside two months," as opined by Satya Nadella of Microsoft.

This change agent of global magnitude is transforming all aspects of human life from workplace, schools, shopping, eating out, entertainment, fitness, healthcare, travel, and much more. Activities that were in the physical realms will become completely or partially virtual, transitioning us to a hybrid "phidigtal" world. It will accelerate some of the trends that were already in motion such as remote working, remote learning, telemedicine, online shopping, virtual gatherings. It will also force some global economies to divert physical infrastructure investments such as highways and buildings toward digital infrastructure that can create the platform for digital acceleration. Organizations and nations that take bold and decisive steps toward digital acceleration are likely to surge ahead of their peers and define the next frontier of the digital economy.

References

1. Forbes, 2,000 COVID-19 scams killed by British Spy Unit in just one month Thomas Brewster, April 20, 2020. Retrieved from: https://www.forbes.com/sites/thomasbrewster/2020/04/20/2000-covid-19-scams-killed-by-british-spy-unit-in-just-one-month/#6e1ff5db34e4
2. Abigail Hess, Google announces 100,000 scholarships for online certificates in data analytics, project management and UX, CNBC, July 13, 2020. Retrieved from: https://www.cnbc.com/2020/07/13/google-announces-certificates-in-data-project-management-and-ux.html
3. Alex McFarland, December 22, 2019, Retrieved from: https://www.unite.ai/intel-acquires-ai-startup-habana/
4. Alibaba delivers strong financial results, cloud revenue climbs 58%, Natalie Gagliordi May 22, 2020, ZDNet. Retrieved from: https://www.zdnet.com/article/alibaba-delivers-strong-financial-results-cloud-revenue-climbs-58/

5. B.F., Why the weekend isn't longer, Sep 21, 2018, Retrieved from: https://www.economist.com/the-economist-explains/2018/09/21/why-the-weekend-isnt-longer?utm_source=Twitter&utm_medium=Economist_Films&utm_campaign=Link_Description&utm_term=&utm_content=&linkId=100000008825541

6. Brie Weiler Reynolds, "FlexJobs 2018 Annual Survey: Workers believe a flexible or remote job can help save money, reduce stress, and more," FlexJobs, September 8, 2018.

7. https://news.arizona.edu/story/university-arizona-launches-global-campus.

8. Catherine Clifford, May 29, 2018. This is Bill Gates' favorite class – and you can take it online for free, Retrieved from: https://www.cnbc.com/2018/05/29/bill-gates-favorite-online-class-big-history-by-david-christian.html

9. CoSo Cloud, "CoSo cloud survey shows working remotely benefits employers and employees," February 17, 2015.

10. ODoc Facebook page, Retrieved from: https://www.facebook.com/odocHQ/posts/we-are-humbled-to-join-hands-with-our-government-doctors-to-launch-the-sri-lanka/2903389216350029/

11. Dougal Shaw, Coronavirus: What's it like to start a new job when working remotely? BBC News, June 17, 2020. Retrieved from: https://www.bbc.com/news/business-52900325

12. Fiona Wilson, *Organizational Behaviour and Work: A Critical Introduction*, OUP Oxford, January 21, 2010, Chapter 2.

13. https://ec.europa.eu/eurostat/web/products-eurostat-news/-/EDN-20181123-1

14. https://www.bighistoryproject.com/home

15. https://www.gartner.com/en/research/methodologies/gartner-hype-cycle

16. https://www.intel.com/content/www/us/en/silicon-innovations/moores-law-technology.html

17. https://www.theedgemarkets.com/article/cover-story-elearning-acceleration

18. https://www.statista.com/statistics/610271/worldwide-personal-computers-installed-base/

19. https://www.oecd.org/future-of-work/#a-world-reshaped-by-digitalisation

20. ILO Press Release. "Covid-19 causes devastating losses in working hours and employment," International Labour Organization, April 7, 2020.

21. Intel Corporation (2012), Fun facts: Exactly how small (and cool) is 22 nanometres? [online]. Available at https://www.intel.com/content/dam/www/public/us/en/documents/corporate-information/history-moores-law-fun-facts-factsheet.pdf/ (Accessed: May 17, 2020).

22. Internet World Stats, Usage and Population Statistics, retrieved from: https://www.internetworldstats.com/stats.htm

23. Ira Kaufman, @ira9201, October 24, 2011, Retrieved from: https://www.socialmediatoday.com/content/are-you-digital-alien-digital-immigrant-or-digital-native-marketing-digital-who

24. Jacob Morgan, The Future of Work: Attract New Talent, *Build Better Leaders, and Create a Competitive Organization*, 1st edition, New Jersey: Wiley (August 25, 2014).

25. Jared Spataro, 2 years of digital transformation in 2 months, Corporate Vice President for Microsoft 365, April 30, 2020. Retrieved from: https://www.microsoft.com/en-us/microsoft-365/blog/2020/04/30/2-years-digital-transformation-2-months/

26. Jared Spataro, Remote work trend report: meetings, Corporate Vice President for Microsoft 365, April 9, 2020, Retrieved from: https://www.microsoft.com/en-us/microsoft-365/blog/2020/04/09/remote-work-trend-report-meetings/

27. Jeff Desjardins, July 6, 2018, Retrieved from: https://www.visualcapitalist.com/visualizing-worlds-20-largest-tech-giants/
28. Karen Hao, China has started a grand experiment in AI education. It could reshape how the world learns, MIT Technology Review, August 2, 2019.
29. Libby Bacon, Sean Morris and Nicole Overley, COVID-19 and the virtualization of government: Responding, recovering, and preparing to thrive in the future of work, Deloitte 28 April 2020. Retrieved from: https://www2.deloitte.com/us/en/insights/economy/covid-19/covid-19-and-the-virtualization-of-government.html
30. Mark Gurman, April 4, 2020, Retrieved from: https://www.bloomberg.com/news/articles/2020-04-03/apple-acquires-ai-startup-to-better-understand-natural-language
31. Mark Gurman, May 14, 2020, Retrieved from: https://www.bloomberg.com/news/articles/2020-05-14/apple-acquires-startup-nextvr-to-gain-virtual-reality-content
32. Mark Minevich, Seeing results from AI, even during Covid-19 recession, Forbes, June 2, 2020, Retrieved from: https://www.forbes.com/sites/markminevich/2020/06/09/seeing-results-from-ai-even-during-covid19-recession
33. Mary Meeker's famous Internet Trends 2018, Kleiner Perkins, Retrieved from: https://www.kleinerperkins.com/perspectives/internet-trends-report-2018/
34. Mary Baker, April 14, 2020, Gartner Press Release, Retrieved from: https://www.gartner.com/en/newsroom/press-releases/2020-04-14-gartner-hr-survey-reveals-41–of-employees-likely-to-
35. Nell Lewis, CNN Business Coronavirus lockdown could give online education a lasting boost in India, Retrieved from: https://edition.cnn.com/2020/04/08/tech/online-education-india-coronavirus-spc/index.html
36. Sooraj Shah, Coronavirus: What's it like to be laid off over Zoom? BBC News, June 2, 2020. Retrieved from: https://www.bbc.com/news/business-52830257
37. OECD (2019), "Education at a glance." Retrieved from: https://read.oecd-ilibrary.org/education/education-at-a-glance-2019_f8d7880d-en#page233
38. Time Well Spent by WSJ and ICSC, Retrieved from: https://partners.wsj.com/icsc/shopping-for-the-truth/time-well-spent/
39. Twitter, Retrieved from: https://twitter.com/mahesh_amalean/status/1267784039689265153
40. UNESCO May 2020, Retrieved from: https://gemreportunesco.wordpress.com/2020/05/15/distance-learning-denied/
41. United States Office of Personnel Management, Status of telework in the Federal government: Report to Congress, fiscal year 2017, January 2019.
42. We've broken down your entire life into years spent doing tasks by Leigh Campbell Huffpost, October 19, 2017, Retrieved from: https://www.huffingtonpost.com.au/2017/10/18/weve-broken-down-your-entire-life-into-years-spent-doing-tasks_
43. Zack Friedman, Student loan debt statistics in 2020: A record $1.6 trillion, Forbes, February 3, 2020, Retrieved from: https://www.forbes.com/sites/zackfriedman/2020/02/03/student-loan-debt-statistics/#b44e30281fef

7 Exacerbating the pandemic?

Assessing the critical role of religious congregations in the Indian subcontinent

Animesh Roul

Introduction

The SARS-CoV-2 (Coronavirus) that encircled the world within weeks of its outbreak in China's Hubei province in late December 2019 has affected over (as of August 01, 2020) 17,409,667 people with 669,753 reported deaths.[1] While the death and infections continues to increase, **it** is now spread to all inhabited continents and affected people irrespective of their color, creed, and character. This unprecedented pandemic has certainly exposed myriad vulnerabilities of **the** modern world, severely questioning so-called human progress in the sphere of scientific innovations and advances in global health care system. It also exposed the socio-religious divide and defiance within communities and lack of collective responsibilities in the face of this gargantuan challenge before the humanity at present. Undoubtedly, this deadly virus spread has occupied center stage in the international and regional security discourse. Amid this unprecedented global calamity, obstinate and opportunistic ultra conservative religious groups willfully resist and defy prescribed norms made to restrict horizontal spread of the deadly pathogen. Similar to the Islamist jihadi forces who have blatantly celebrated the deaths and destruction due to the spread of the disease terming the virus as "divine solider" or "divine retribution," several mainstream but orthodox religious institutions observed the virus as a God-sent force and it is playing havoc due to widespread disobedience to God and increasing human sins on this earth. These conservative religious groups and sub-groups (Muslim, Jewish, and Christian) have invoked eschatological belief such as "Day of Judgement" to justify it as "God given phenomena" and "He" only can help the humanity from this disaster and prayer is the last resort for survival.[2] These groups and their spiritual leaders showed irresponsible behavior and sometimes willful negligence to exacerbate the virus spread, complicating the fight against the pandemic with their superstitions and blind believe in their respective supreme entities.

Termed often as "super-spreader" or "virus multiplier," they have violated pandemic specific health guidelines by international and national bodies and defied the laws of the land by invoking God's law to protect the believers or faithful. Examples are aplenty, starting from the fringe Shincheonji Church of Jesus in Degu (South Korea) whose messianic leader Lee Man-hee termed the virus as

DOI: 10.4324/9781003197416-7

the "devil" and banned protective masks during prayers in late February 2020. Later a surge of coronavirus infections in the country was traced to gatherings at this Church.[3] Similarly, in India and Pakistan, the transnational Islamic pietist group Tablighi Jamaat's Delhi and Lahore congregations in early March 2020 proved to be COVID-19 super-spreader event venues due to non-compliance of government's pandemic orders.

Amid the unprecedented pandemic situation, recalcitrant religious congregations have surfaced everywhere contributing negatively and jeopardizing the collective battle against the COVID-19 pandemic. Though not every time, these groups or their ideologues were at fault. At times there was government negligence in allowing prayer meetings or allowing devotees or adherents to engage in regular rituals (e.g. the Christian Open Door prayers in France) to have contributed to some extent in the virus spread. Also at times, the infected people of particular religions have spread the virus when they resumed regular religious rituals even with pandemic specific measures in place. In India, several employees of a major Hindu temple tested positive for COVID-19 after the temple was opened for pilgrims in early June, 2020 following relaxation of lockdown restrictions (Hindustan Times, August 10).[4] However, Tablighi Jamaat received much attention in South Asia for its congregations defying the COVID-19 guidelines in both Pakistan and India during the initial phase of the pandemic. Termed as a COVID-19 "accelerator" and "super-spreader," the group and its adherents were blamed for collective ignorance or defiance of "man-made" pandemic laws. Religious leaders and groups disregarded the fact that mass confluence of people in close proximities might prove to be fertile ground for any viral respiratory infection. Indeed, mass religious gatherings across Asia triggered coronavirus spread and exacerbated the pandemic wave.

This paper highlights the controversial, rather critical role of religious and faith-based congregations in South Asian region, especially in India, Pakistan, Sri Lanka, and Bangladesh in transmitting or spreading the virus, either intentionally or inadvertently defying pandemic specific regulations. Fortunately, Bangladesh escaped unscathed from COVID-19 spike due to large gatherings but the rest of the three countries of South Asia have experienced more or less COVID-19 spike due to the unrestricted and sometimes deliberate religious gatherings or congregations that exacerbated the COVID-19 cases substantially and even proved fatal. The paper also examines how these communities, religious groups, and institutions practice of group activities defying government directives of lockdown and social distancing have accelerated virus transmissions and compromised safety and security of others.

India

In India, Tablighi Jamaat (hereafter, TJ or Jamaat), a transnational ultra-conservative proselytizing group borne out of the larger Deoband movement of Northern India, caught all the attention during the height of the emerging COVID crisis in early 2020.[5] A two-day TJ congregation event in Delhi's

Nizamuddin area came under severe criticism when its Delhi-based leaders organized a mass gathering of around 4,500 people from India and abroad despite the looming COVID-19 crisis on the horizon. It also came under disparagement for housing hundreds of Jamaat member preachers in its headquarters in Delhi even after the scheduled event, defying pandemic restrictions. Their refusal to suspend the gatherings could lead to potential widespread dispersal of infections.

The TJ's international executive committee meeting (*Aalami Mashwara*) was scheduled on March 8–10, 2020[6] while two other regional branch meets were scheduled subsequently in South Eastern State of Andhra Pradesh[7] and Tamil Nadu between March 15 and March 24.[8] These meetings usually attract less numbers of members than TJ's International Conclave (*Aalami Ijtima*) which usually is attended by thousands of people across the country and abroad. Sometime before the COVID-19 infection spread and subsequent preventive measures and restrictions were undertaken, the Jamaat had organized its international conclave at Brahmbarada, Jajpur district between February 29 and March 02 in Eastern India's Odisha state.[9] Later, many of those attending the Jajpur Conclave traveled to the National Capital New Delhi to attend the subsequent meetings along with newly arrived attendees. However, the most plausible source of initial virus infections could be the Tablighi gathering in Malaysia held between February 27 and March 3. Several of Kuala Lumpur attendees have traveled to South Asia for subsequent events in New Delhi and in Lahore, Pakistan (discussed later in the chapter).[10]

Foreigners mostly from Thailand, Nepal, Myanmar, Sri Lanka, Indonesia, Bangladesh, Malaysia, and Kyrgyzstan participated in all these TJ's meetings and congregations, including New Delhi's Nizamuddin event. Several of these foreign nationals had six-month tourist visas. According to one Indian government source, over 2,000 foreigners from 70 countries arrived in India since January 1, 2020 to participate in Tablighi Jamaat's various activities and over 1,000 were stranded at Nizamuddin due to the COVID-19 lockdown. TJ's New Delhi events were organized despite the local government's order issued on March 13, 2020 prohibiting large gatherings and assembly. The organizers of TJ meetings may have taken the COVID-19 alerts lightly or miscalculated the coming lockdowns and strict social distancing restrictions. Possibly unaware of the presence of coronavirus among them already, the TJ organizers ignored these guidelines and flouted the norms imposed for the looming contagion. It continued with the congregation of preachers in the famed Banglewali Masjid (TJ's headquarters, also known as the "Markaz") in Nizamuddin, New Delhi as per their schedule.

The alert about TJ's congregations and fear of possible spread of coronavirus through the traveling preachers amid the COVID-19 situation in India surfaced for the first time when an Indonesian was tested positive with coronavirus on March 18. He had participated in the Delhi congregation and was traveling to Telangana, located in eastern India. The Internal Affair Ministry alerted all state governments about these traveling preachers of the TJ on March 21. Soon, the Telangana authorities reported at least 10 Indonesians had tested positive for coronavirus in Karimnagar.[11] In Delhi, at least 24 attendees were initially found to be COVID-19 positive as civic authorities cleared and sanitized the TJ's headquarters which emerged as an epicenter for the coronavirus spread in the capital and elsewhere in the country. By the end of March, the local civic and health authorities sent about 2,300 inmates to hospital wards and quarantines. According to the government release of early April 2020, nearly 400 positive cases detected across ten states and Union Territories had links to the Tablighi Jamaat cluster in Delhi's Nizamuddin. The release also added that out of nearly 2,000 Tablighi Jamaat members in Delhi, 1,804 were quarantined while 334 had been admitted to different hospitals.[12]

In mid-April 2020, the government released a statement underscoring how the TJ organizers and followers defied the strict lockdown norms and social distancing restrictions that added misery to the ongoing pandemic mitigation efforts. It categorically noted that nearly 29.8% of the country's total COVID-19 cases (which was approximately 14,378 cases at that time) were linked to the Nizamuddin Markaz where TJ preachers were staying during the events and in the lockdown period. According to the information shared by the Ministry of Health and Family Welfare, the attendees of the congregation infected others in 23 states and union territories.[13] It also added that the Delhi congregations had direct connection with the spike in COVID-19 cases in the other states. Of the total cases in Tamil Nadu, 84% were linked to the Tablighi Jamaat event, making it the most affected state, Telangana 79%, followed by Delhi at 63%, Andhra Pradesh (61%), and Uttar Pradesh (59%).[14] Similarly, in Jammu and Kashmir, 25 COVID-19 cases were detected on April 13, 2020 and among them, 12 persons had Tablighi Jamaat connection.

The TJ was also caught in a web of alleged illegal activities that usually went unnoticed in the past. The foreign nationals who had attended the TJ events were investigated and charge sheets were filed against them for attending the religious congregation at Nizamuddin Markaz by violating visa conditions, indulging in missionary activities illegally and violating government's pandemic specific guidelines issued in the wake of COVID-19 outbreak in the country. In June 2020, Delhi police filed 59 charge sheets, including supplementaries, against 956 foreigners belonging to 36 different countries in the case. As of mid-July, some 532 foreigners who faced charge sheets from 34 countries received bail. Among them 98 members were Indonesians, 82 from Kyrgyzstan and 80 from Bangladesh. According to the charge sheets, all the foreigners were booked for violation of visa rules, guidelines issued in the wake of COVID-19 pandemic, Epidemic Diseases Act, Disaster Management Act, and prohibitory orders under Section 144 of Code of Criminal Procedure. They were also booked for the offenses under Sections 188 (Disobedience to order duly promulgated by public servant), 269 (Negligent act likely to spread infection of disease dangerous to life), 270 (Malignant act likely to spread infection of disease dangerous to life) and 271 (Disobedience to quarantine rule) of the Indian Penal Code (IPC).[15]

The TJ leader Maulana Mohammad Saad Kandhlawi was blamed for negligence and for violation of the Epidemic Diseases Act (EDA-1897).[16] The Delhi

Police had booked him and several other congregation organizers under the Epidemic Act 1897 and under different sections of the IPC for violation of government directions given to the management of TJ Markaz in Nizamuddin regarding restriction of social, political, and religious gathering and for not taking health and hygiene-related safety measures, including social distancing. Denying any transgression, the Jamaat leadership claimed that due to sudden announcement of "Janata Curfew"[17] on March 22, followed by a three-week national lockdown starting from March 24, hundreds of Jamaat members were stranded at the Markaz itself while about 1,500 had left for their destinations. Even though the Prime Minister of India announced this experimental limited lockdown and the subsequent pan-India lockdown within a few days gaps, the Jamaat leaders failed to inform or communicate with the concerned authorities regarding the stranded inmates at its headquarters.

Investigating agencies claimed that Saad and his team failed to advise the event participants in accordance with government's guidelines for the prevention and treatment of the novel coronavirus. Saad and his team were found to be communicating with TJ members either directly or through indirect means such as audio messages, exhorting or encouraging them not to panic and not to leave the mosque. A cursory look at Saad Kandhlawi's controversial and sometime confusing speeches during the initial days of lockdown conveys the group's non-compliance and irresponsible behaviors, even though the TJ garnered sympathies from members of the society due to media backlash following the rise of COVID cases. The spiritual leader's statements to it members invoking God's wrath narratives and encouraging assembly at mosques for prayers by not heeding to government health guidelines can be found in speeches delivered on March 20, 22, and 25. These three speeches were related to the looming COVID-19 situation in the country and also reflect how the spiritual leader of TJ defied the rules initially but tried to abide by the pandemic guidelines when things got out of hand.[18]

On March 22, Saad Kandhlawi underscored the pandemic-specific guidelines of social distance and non-assembly as "false remedial measures." He said in his audio speech that "It's a false belief the disease spreads through assembling in the mosques [...] these people (government bodies) perceive dangers in Namaz. Allah has brought the calamity as a punishment for leaving the mosques, and they think they can ward off the calamity by leaving the mosque. Think over it. How ridiculous!" He further said, "Satan is using this opportunity as it has always done to lead us astray from our religious duties in the name of precautions, treatment and protection. Whenever a calamity strikes, Satan makes the victims of calamity commit such acts which destroy their rewards and add to their woes. This is the time to populate the mosques and to invite the ummah toward repentance."[19]

However, on March 25, Saad changed his tone and tenor of his speech urging TJ followers to take the government's directives and doctors' advice as these are not against Islam and Shari'a or also not against the principles of the Dawah and Tabligh. He emphasized not to compromise or sacrifice religious duties.

The Indian government was also conscious about the fact that there was a growing discontent against the TJ that spiraled into a larger anti-Muslim wave triggering a polarized discourse in India. Coupled with social media misinformation, not only Tablighi adherents, but the whole Muslim community faced social backlash as the Jamaat-linked cases came to surface. The TJ leaders and the preachers were labeled as "super-spreaders" for three reasons: Their failure to report the infections to the authority, due to the obstinate behavior toward obeying pandemic orders and initial non-cooperation with civic and medical authorities. However, the authorities in Delhi urged not to brand a community (i.e. Muslims in particular) and locations (e.g. Nizamuddin Markaz) as epicenters or hotspots for the COVID-19 spread. It also issued notice underscoring the spread of any misinformation or exaggeration of certain events relating to the Tablighi preachers and intentional proliferations of coronavirus. It is also imperative to note, larger Muslim minorities of India abided the pandemic guidelines and followed or cooperated with authorities.

Apart from the Tablighi Jamaat events in New Delhi and elsewhere, which contributed to a nation-wide spike in COVID-19 cases, there were cases of negligence that surfaced associated with other (Hindu, Jain, and Sikh) religious gatherings or congregations that took place during the early months of the outbreak. It is true that while TJ's negligence and irresponsible actions triggered community-specific criticism, backlash, and discrimination, other similar violations by other religious groups were hardly highlighted nor received as much attention primarily due to the low number of COVID-19 infections they caused or localized effect of the transgression.

A Sikh preacher named Baldev Singh, who had a travel history to Italy and Germany, was found to be responsible for infecting several of his followers in Punjab. He defied the pandemic restriction and violated his compulsory home quarantine order after his return to India. He attended the Hola Mohalla festival, a three-day long Sikh festival on March 10–12, held at Anandpur city and offered his blessings to his followers and even visited their homes. He died along with his two fellow associates on March 18 due to COVID-19. Later it was found that out of the first 33 positive cases in Punjab state in North India, 23 were directly linked to this Sikh preacher.

On May 13, hundreds of people gathered to welcome the Jain saint (Digambar sect) Praman Sagar who visited Banda city in Sagar, Madhya Pradesh. The saint was traveling along with his retinue. The visual of the event showed that devotees did not follow social distancing norm or compulsory use of mask guidelines as they descended to the city street to welcome the Jain saint and his team. A case was registered against hundreds of unidentified people for violation of preventive orders issued during countrywide lockdown (New Indian Express, May 13).[20] Though there was no evidence of a COVID-19 spike in the district, the saint himself urged people later not to defy pandemic orders to prevent the virus spread, as it comes under moral duty of every citizen, irrespective of his/her religious beliefs.

In mid-April 2020, another violation came to notice in Karnataka's Rawoor village in Gulbarga district, when hundreds of Hindu devotees participated in Siddhalingeswara chariot festival, violating COVID-19 lockdown restrictions. Earlier, the district was considered to be the most infected with coronavirus and the first COVID-19 death was reported from Gulbarga on March 12.[21] After a wave of social media coverage of that violation, a case was registered against 20 people and the temple management under Sections 188, 143, 269 of the IPC. At least five organizers of the Siddalingeshwara fair were arrested for violating the lockdown.

Although the larger Christian community of India cooperated well with the government orders and pandemic restrictions, a Catholic Church in Kerala came on the radar when its chief priest Poly Padayattil led a Sunday Mass in Nithya Sahaya Matha (Mother of Perpetual Help) church at Koodapuzha in Thrissur district, violating state directives. On March 22, at the Koodappuzha Mass, hundreds of people attended the function. The chief priest and several people who attended the ceremony were identified and cases were registered against them subsequently.[22] Earlier Kerala Police had booked two other Catholic priests for conducting mass meetings with hundreds of people in attendance despite strict direction to suspend all religious gatherings and services in the wake of COVID-19 in Kasaragod district. Thomas Pattamkulam, the vicar of St Joseph Forane Church at Kollichal in Panathady and his assistant vicar Joseph Orath were booked by the local police for endangering public health. They were charged with IPC Section 188 (Disobeying order passed by public servant and which can cause danger to human life, health or safety) and Section 269 (negligent act likely to spread infection of disease dangerous to life).[23]

Again on March 29, police arrested ten people, including two Catholic priests and three nuns in Chettappalam, near Mananthavady in Wayanad district for celebrating Sunday Mass, defying pandemic specific prohibitory orders. The incident happened when the country was witnessing the 21-day of pan-India lockdown.[24]

Unlike the TJ's congregation in New Delhi, all the other abovementioned religious congregations representing different religions and faiths that defied pandemic norms were not found to be conducting super-spreader events. But these different religious groups and individuals have clearly flouted the pandemic laws and restrictions imposed to contain the spread of the virus during the heights of the outbreak. When the pandemic-related restrictions and lockdown were relaxed or partially lifted post-July 2020, religious activities in India resumed with all safety norms in place.

Pakistan

The COVID-19 pandemic swept through Pakistan, the second most affected country in South Asia since late February 2020. However, the real effect of the virus was felt around mid-March when the infective cases increased and pandemic-specific restriction such as lockdown and social distancing norms were implemented. Similar to India, the Tablighi Jamaat group had a major role in exacerbating the COVID-19 cases in Pakistan too. Another example of blatant defiance of the law of the land and ignorance toward the looming calamity made the COVID-19 situation in Pakistan complicated. Like India, TJ Pakistan's religious congregation turned out to be a major COVID-19 super spreader event.

Tablighi Jamaat, Lahore

Jamaat's controversial congregation that took place in its Raiwind Markaz (headquarters) in Lahore, Punjab province, came under scanner as the epicenter of COVID-19 infection. A five-day international conclave (*Aalami ijtima*) was held starting March 10, amid the pandemic fears. Thousands of Islamic scholars and preachers from Pakistan and different parts of the world attended this congregation. About 3,000 Islamic preachers and scholars from 40 countries, including the United States, Europe, and South East Asian countries descended to Lahore for this annual congregation. According to media reports, the provincial government's request for the post-ponement of the conclave due to the COVID-19 was rejected by the TJ leadership. However, later the event was cut short and ended on March 12 with the federal government's intervention.

Within weeks, the Punjab health department reported that over 1,100 Tablighi Jamaat members tested positive for coronavirus in the Punjab province. The traveling preachers also took the infection to other parts of the country. However, the foreign nationals were unable to return to their home destinations due to imposition of countrywide lockdown and abrupt stopping of all international flight operations. The sprawling Raiwind headquarters (Markaz) soon turned into a quarantined center for the stranded Jamaat members as situation worsened in the country. Large number of positive cases were reported from Raiwind Markaz turning the TJ headquarters into an epicenter of COVID-19 with 404 confirmed cases.[25] A senior TJ member, Maulana Suhaib Rumi (head of Faisalabad chapter), died of the virus. Media reports said that in early week of April 2020, around 20,000 people who attended the event have been quarantined, as a massive contact tracing operation was undertaken by the Punjab authorities.[26] Even though several congregation attendees were tracked down across the country and placed in quarantine centers, the infection had already gone out of hand by then. According to an estimation released on April 18, out of several thousands of confirmed COVID-19 patients in Pakistan, there were 1,352 TJ members in Punjab itself. Further, a location wise data showed how the contagion spread across Punjab province using TJ members as vector. Out of the 1,352 confirmed TJ cases, 577 were reported from Raiwind Markaz, 121 from Sargodha, 118 from Multan, 62 from Bhakkar, 61 from Muzaffargarh, 45 from Rahim Yar Khan, 41 from Jhelum, 37 from Vehari, 35 in Hafizabad, 34 in Bahawalpur, 31 in Layyah, 23 in Khushab, 22 in Narowal, 19 in Sialkot, 18 in Faisalabad, 17 in Mandi Bahauddin, 16 in Rawalpindi, 14 in Gujrat, 13 in Bahawalnagar, 12 in Sheikhupura, 10 in Gujranwala, nine in Rajanpur, seven each in Mianwali and Sahiwal and two cases from Nankana

Sahib.[27] Subsequently, the number of COVID-19 infection directly linked to the Raiwind congregation reached 2,258, accounting for around 27% of the country's total cases. At that time, Pakistan's total coronavirus patients were recorded at 9,565 with nearly 200 deaths.[28]

Earlier in April, a massive manhunt was launched to trace the TJ preachers who had attended the Raiwind event. Over 5,000 search teams were formed each comprising eight members to search and sweep through mosque's spread across Pakistan.[29]

The Tablighi Jamaat's controversial congregation was criticized by the Science and Technology Minister Fawad Chaudhry who blamed Jamaat's leadership and their decision to organize the conclave against the government's advice. He expressed his displeasure on social media that outbreak has spread in Pakistan due to the ignorance of this religious group.[30] However, the TJ members and its leaders remained defiant against the government's pandemic restrictions and media backlash against the group. Some of its top leaders criticized the media vilification of the Tablighi Jamaat, and said that any action against preachers' would invite God's wrath. Many Jamaat leaders such as Maulana Tariq Jameel termed the pandemic itself as "God's wrath" and urged people to seek God's forgiveness to ward off the disease. He even went a step further on a live TV debate and made a shocking remark that scantily dressed women were responsible for this wrath as well. He later, however, retracted and urged his followers to exercise caution and adopt preventive measures.[31]

Shia Pilgrims from Iran

During the initial phase of the outbreak, the majority of Pakistan's COVID-19 cases were the result of the returning Shia pilgrims (known as Zaireen) from neighboring Iran, through the Taftan (Balochistan) border, where the coronavirus was at its peak at that time and the country was the second worst-hit Asian country after China. Those who visited Iranian cities like Qom and Mashad were primarily infected with the virus. Out of the total 2,039 confirmed cases in Pakistan till April 1, 46% had a travel history to Iran. In Balochistan, 145 out of 190 confirmed cases and in Gilgit Baltistan 170 out of 210 cases were returnees from Iran.[32] In Punjab, the spread of virus with a Iranian link was worst with 701 confirmed patients identified. Among them, 457 cases were reported from Multan, 221 from Dera Ghazi Khan, and 23 in Faisalabad of Punjab province.[33] However, the government's swift and forceful action at the borders somehow restricted the spread of the virus to some extent by quarantining the pilgrims. Even though these cases are linked directly to religious pilgrimage and the virus affected a particular sect of Islam, these cluster of COVID-19 cases were unlike TJ cluster. The Shia pilgrims were to be blamed along with the government for their incompetence at the outset of pandemic. The pilgrims as such did not defy any pandemic laws during the initial period of the outbreak in Pakistan rather it was the government's mishandling that caused a deteriorating situation at the border.

Other than TJ COVID clusters, there were conservative and recalcitrant Islamic clerics who not only defended TJ's wrong-doings and negligence, but also criticized government orders to close down mosques and collective Friday prayers. Defying pandemic directives, those mosques which allowed congregational prayers later turned out to be the virus spreaders. The famed Red Mosque (Lal Lasjid) in the capital Islamabad led this anti-COVID-19 bandwagon clearly flouting pandemic laws and opened its gate for huge prayer gatherings. Earlier, the leader of Red Mosque told *Al Jazeera* that "Lockdowns are not the answer to these problems [...] the people should not be made to fear things right now, they should have faith in God at this time, and to place their hope in him ... If death is written for you, then it will come."[34] Subsequently, Pakistan's authorities allowed mosque prayers knowing very well that the Islamic practices such as prayers in mosques remain a sensitive issue in the country. Initially, it stipulated mosque gatherings to a maximum of five people, but that provoked strong reactions from Islamic clerics and scholars.[35] Later more relaxations were granted for congregational prayers with strict social distancing and other COVID-19 measures. In view of religious sensitivity in the month of Ramadan, under the stewardship of the president of Pakistan, both the government and Islamic cleric bodies' recommendations were approved as a 20-point action plan as a standard operating procedure for prayers and limited gatherings in the mosques.[36]

There is a general discontent, however, that remains within the larger civil society in Pakistan about the opening of mosque congregations amid the threat of COVID-19. The government also faced criticism for acting under duress and succumbing to the pressure from conservative religious lobbies that had shown a lack of discipline and contempt for the rule of the land at the first place.

Bangladesh

Bangladesh, the other South Asian country, also witnessed massive COVID-19 infections and the government imposed a complete lockdown on March 24, 2020 to break the chain of the contagion. Prior to the lockdown, the virus reached Bangladesh with confirmed cases on March 8 when three people arrived from Italy, the worst affected country in Europe by then. The civic authorities in Bangladesh then restricted mass gatherings, including mosque congregations as a preventive measure against the spread of COVID-19.

Khatme Shifa Mass Prayer

Despite the COVID preventive measures in place, nearly 25,000 people descended on the streets to participate in a special prayer session known as "Khatme Shifa" for protection against coronavirus.[37] The gathering was organized at the Central Eidghah in Raipur town, located in Lakshmipur district of Chittagong division on March 18. The prayer was led by Chittagong's Andarkilla Shahi Jama Mosque chief Maolana Syed Anwar Hossain and organized by Haiderganj Taheria Central Eidgah Jama Mosque.[38] Islamic believers chanted these healing verses from the Qur'an to save the country from the looming pandemic on the horizon. It caught the district authorities off guard as the organizers did not have the necessary government permission for this massive gathering. The event was vehemently criticized by media and civil society across the spectrum at a time when the country was preparing for the pandemic challenges ahead. The organizers of this event, however, admitted the unexpected turn outs and regretted the event following the government and law enforcement's interventions. Though the prayer and massive gathering did not cause any spike in Coronavirus cases in Chittagong, ironically enough, on the day of mass prayer at Lakhmipur, Bangladesh, the first COVID-19 death was reported. By the end of March 2020, the country had over 50 confirmed cases with five deaths. By mid-July 2020, the number of confirmed COVID cases crossed 200,000 with 2,500 deaths.[39]

Sri Lanka

Sri Lanka has a relatively low number of COVID-19 cases in comparison to its northern neighbors, with around 2,700 confirmed cases and 11 deaths by mid-July 2020. Although the reasons behind the lower number of cases were assigned to less testing, the teardrop island nation of South Asia too witnessed similar religious congregations that became a hurdle in the fight against the coronavirus.

Philadelphia Missionary Church, Jaffna

During the initial phase of the pandemic, on March 15, 2020, the visiting evangelist pastor of Philadelphia Missionary Church in Kandy Road, Ariyalai, Jaffna urged his followers in the Northern Province to attend his mass supposedly for containment of the coronavirus. The pastor of the church, a Switzerland-based Sri Lankan national Paul Satkunarajah, led the prayer gathering which was attended by 240 people where pandemic specific norms of social distance were openly flouted. He reportedly hugged and gave his blessings to the people at the congregation. Subsequently, he was found corona positive and reportedly he had traveled back to (his adopted country) Switzerland for treatment. Among the people who attended the mass with Paul Satkunarajah, seven people were found to be infected with COVID-19 while others were quarantined by the authorities for a stipulated period of time.[40] Following this incident, Sri Lankan authorities took steps to monitor the visiting evangelist missionaries and considered them as a roadblock in the battle against COVID-19.

Concluding Observations

The World Health Organization (WHO) issued guidelines (though lately) in April 2020 against any sort of collective prayers or gatherings in the name of religion and urged religious leaders and organizations to follow the guidelines.[41]

The "social distancing" which has been part of primary preventive strategy for virus spread has been implemented. The WHO also warned that any mass gathering in close approximation could trigger a spread of the virus and any refusal to adhere to these guidelines could lead to potential widespread dispersal of infections. However, much before this WHO warning, several unrestricted mobilization and gatherings in early weeks of this pandemic, mostly in the first three months of the pandemic (March–April–May) spread, proved to be the principal points for virus dispersal across South Asia. Even though, in the subsequent months (June–July–August), when the strict pandemic norms were relaxed, the virus continued to affect religious gatherings and pilgrim centers sporadically either due to defiance and negligence or complacency about the COVID-19 virulence.

The COVID-19 pandemic has proved that the virus has infected people most who had a travel history and that condition triggered global, local, and community transmissions. While the air and sea route leisure and business travel played a measure role in spreading the virus across the world, religious gatherings of faithful and subsequent traveling and mixing with new populations contributed substantially to the virus spread. It is an established fact that religious groups encourage and prescribe mass mobilization of faithful devotees and community congregations of its followers as part of their core rituals. However, organizing religious congregations amid a looming threat of an infectious pandemic is nothing but a crime and negligence, suggesting irresponsibility and utter disregard to "man-made" laws and norms. Several instances discussed in this chapter proved that these congregations were in outright defiance and hinderance when authorities were struggling to mitigate the larger health and security challenges.

When governments in South Asia were taking measures to contain the COVID-19 spread, the lack of people's cooperation, irrespective of their religious orientations complicated the process to a large extent. These groups of adherents considered government's pandemic measures such as prohibitions on congregations, social distance, closure of worship, and prayer places as an imposition on their freedom of religion and also a challenge to their respective Gods. However, largely though the foregoing religious groups in particular suffered backlash for their non-compliance with the Pandemic laws, they have not subjected to persecution or harassment either in India, Pakistan or in Sri Lanka. Rather, their disregard for the laws of the land and initial defiance, earned them hateful messaging restricted only to social and mainstream media. Even these groups were criticized by their own community members due to their careless attitude toward the disease mitigation. Indeed, some of these religious gatherings and mass prayers have emerged as a virus multiplier during the initial phase of the pandemic as well creating impediments to efforts to mitigate the pandemic.

Notes

1. WHO Coronavirus Disease (COVID-19) Dashboard, August 01, 2020, https://covid19.who.int (Accessed on August 02, 2020).

2. The concept of Judgment Day is a fundamental tenet of Islam that marks the end of the present world. On this day, human beings will be resurrected and judged by their act of righteousness and sinfulness. Accordingly, they will be rewarded "heaven" or "hellfire." See, Juan e Campo, *Encyclopedia of Islam*, Facts on File Inc., New York, 2009, pp. 413–414.

3. Rosie Perper, "A South Korean doomsday church linked to thousands of coronavirus cases is being sued for $82 million in damages," *Insider*, June 25, 2020, https://www.insider.com/south-korea-doomsday-church-shincheonji-sued-daegu-coronavirus-damages-2020-6. Also, see "Coronavirus: In South Korea, mounting anger, rumours over Shincheonji church as cases rise," *SCMP*, February 27, 2020, https://www.scmp.com/week-asia/health-environment/article/3052550/south-korea-mounting-anger-rumours-over-shincheonji

4. "743 Tirupati temple staff tested Covid-19 positive since June 11," *Hindustan Times*, August 10, 2020, https://www.hindustantimes.com/india-news/743-tirupati-temple-staff-tested-covid-19-positive-since-june-11/story-SYypz-RzdlqPh0xdH1ULgyM.html

5. Tablighi Jamaat (preaching party/society) is a prominent Islamic revivalist group representing Sunni Muslim community. It has origins in Mewat city of Haryana State in Northern India. The group was founded nearly 100 years ago by Deobandi Islamic scholar Maulana Muhammad Ilyas Khandhalawi. TJ largely considers the modern world is in a state of ignorance and the movement broadly attempts to bring about a change by infusing its followers with Islamic values and practices. The group is essentially conservative in outlook and orientation, with a strong aversion to rational sciences. See, Animesh Roul, "Transnational Islam in India: Movements, Networks, and Conflict Dynamics," in Peter Mandaville (et al.), *Transnational Islam in South and Southeast Asia: Movements, Networks, and Conflict Dynamics*, National Bureau of Asian Research, Seattle, 2009, pp. 101–120.

6. "Aalami Mashwara 2020," March 8–10, http://www.delhimarkaz.com/p/aalami-mashwara-2020.html (Accessed on June 15, 2020).

7. "Beemari Ka Khauf," Andhra Pradesh Jod 2020, March 17, 2020, http://www.delhimarkaz.com/p/aalami-mashwara-2020.html (Accessed on June 15, 2020).

8. "Musalmano Par Musibaten Aati Rahengi," Tamil Nadu Jod 2020, http://www.delhimarkaz.com/p/aalami-mashwara-2020.html (Accessed on June 15, 2020).

9. "Odisha Alami Ijtima," February 29–March 02, http://www.delhimarkaz.com/p/odisha-ijtima-2020.html (Accessed on June 15, 2020).

10. Sayed A. Quadri, "COVID-19 and religious congregations: Implications for spread of novel pathogens," *International Journal of Infectious Diseases*, No 96, 2020, pp. 219–221. doi:10.1016/j.ijid.2020.05.007.

11. "Centre and Telangana at loggerheads over congregation in capital," *Times of India*, April 03, 2020, http://timesofindia.indiatimes.com/articleshow/74957507.cms?utm_source=contentofinterest&utm_medium=text&utm_campaign=cppst (Accessed on July 18, 2020).

12. "Tablighi explosion: Active Covid-19 cases rise to 1,860; 53 dead," *South Asia Monitor/Indo Asian News Service*, April 03, 2020. https://southasiamonitor.org/index.php/india/tablighi-explosion-active-covid-19-cases-rise-1860-53-dead

13. "30% of India's Covid-19 positive caseload linked to Tablighi Jamaat meet, says govt," *The Print*, April 18, 2020, https://theprint.in/health/30-of-indias-covid-19-positive-caseload-linked-to-tablighi-jamaat-meet-says-govt/404426/

14. "Of the 14,378 COVID-19 infections, 4,291 cases linked to Tablighi Jamaat in Delhi: Health Ministry," *New Indian Express*, https://www.newindianexpress.com/nation/2020/apr/18/of-the-14378-covid-19-infections-4291-cases-linked-to-tablighi-jamaat-in-delhi-health-ministry-2131987.html

15. "Tablighi Jamaat: Delhi court grants bail to 85 Kyrgyzstan nationals," *Economic Times*, July 13, 2020. For more on this, see, "Tablighi Jamaat: Police files charge sheet against 69 foreigners from 9 countries," *Outlook India*, July 28, 2020, https://www.outlookindia.com/newsscroll/tablighi-jamaat-police-files-charge-sheet-against-69-foreigners-from-9-countries/1904622

16. The Epidemic Diseases Act, 1897, which provides for the prevention of the spread of dangerous epidemic diseases, is amended during the ongoing COVID-19 pandemic situation. The Epidemic Diseases (Amendment) Ordinance, 2020, was promulgated on April 22, 202. The Ordinance amends the Act to include protections for healthcare personnel combatting epidemic diseases and expands the powers of the central government to prevent the spread of such diseases. For more information, see *PRS Legislative Research*, April 22, 2020, https://www.prsindia.org/billtrack/epidemic-diseases-amendment-ordinance-2020

17. "What is 'Janta Curfew' and how it will play out," *Hindustan Times*, March 20, 2020, https://www.hindustantimes.com/india-news/what-is-janta-curfew-and-how-it-will-be-implemented/story-YI9fiXNtPpNpzoaXOAELhM.html

18. "Tablighi Jamaat Emir Maulana Mohammad Saad opposes social distancing during coronavirus epidemic, says: 'The Satan Is Using This Opportunity ... To Lead Us Astray from Our Religious Duties In The Name Of Precautions, Treatment, And Protection,'" *MEMRI*, April 06, 2020, https://www.memri.org/reports/tablighi-jamaat-emir-maulana-mohammad-saad-opposes-social-distancing-during-coronavirus#_ednref5

19. Ibid.

20. "Social distancing norms flouted as crowd gathers to greet monks in Madhya Pradesh," *New Indian Express*, May 13, 2020, https://www.newindianexpress.com/nation/2020/may/13/social-distancing-norms-flouted-as-crowd-gathers-to-greet-monk-in-madhya-pradesh-2142866.html

21. "Man from Saudi Arabia dies in Karnataka," *The Telegraph*, March 11, https://www.telegraphindia.com/india/man-from-saudi-arabia-dies-in-karnataka/cid/1752851

22. "Priest held for violating orders by conducting mass," *Kerala Kaumudi*, March 23, 2020, https://keralakaumudi.com/en/news/news.php?id=269022&u=priest-held-for-violating-orders-by-conducting-mass

23. "COVID-19: Two Catholic priests booked in Kerala for violating orders by conducting mass," *Indian Express*, March 19, 2020, https://www.newindianexpress.com/states/kerala/2020/mar/19/covid-19-two-catholic-priests-booked-in-kerala-for-violating-orders-by-conducting-mass-2118977.html

24. "Priests and Nuns arrested," *The Hindu*, March 29, 2020, https://www.thehindu.com/news/national/kerala/priests-nuns-arrested/article31200913.ece

25. "101 preachers among 141 more Covid-19 patients in Lahore," *Dawn*, April 03, 2020, https://www.dawn.com/news/1545940; Also, see "Tableeghi Jamaat in hot water in Pakistan too for Covid-19 spread," *Dawn*, April 08, 2020, https://www.dawn.com/news/1547354

26. "Pakistan quarantines 20,000 following Tabligh gathering in Lahore," *Al Jazeera*, April 06, 2020, https://www.aljazeera.com/news/2020/04/pakistan-quarantines-20000-tabligh-gathering-lahore-200406075221220.html

27. The locations in the list suggest how the virus has reached all corners of Pakistan's largest province with traveling TJ preachers. See, "Corona cases in Pakistan witness sharp increase," *The News*, April 18, 2020, https://www.thenews.com.pk/print/646072-corona-cases-in-pakistan-witness-sharp-increase

28. "27% of Pakistan's Covid-19 cases linked to Raiwind Ijtima: Report," *Express Tribune*, April 21, 2020, https://tribune.com.pk/story/2203599/27-pakistans-covid-19-cases-linked-raiwind-ijtima-report

29. "COVID-19: Search for 41,000 Tableeghi Jamaat members underway," *Geo TV News*, April 02, 2020, https://www.geo.tv/latest/280573-covid-19-search-for-410000-tablighi-jamaat-members-underway

30. "Coronavirus spreads in Pakistan due to ignorance of reactionary religious class: Fawad Chaudhry," *BOL News*, March 26, 2020, https://www.bolnews.com/pakistan/2020/03/coronavirus-spreads-in-pakistan-due-to-ignorance-of-reactionary-religious-class-fawad-chaudhry/

31. "Maulana Tariq Jameel tenders apology over 'slip of tongue,'," *Dawn*, April 25, 2020, https://www.dawn.com/news/1552038

32. "46% Pakistanis with coronavirus have travel history to Iran — WHO," *Arab News*, April 05, 2020, https://www.arabnews.pk/node/1653006/pakistan

33. "Corona cases in Pakistan witness sharp increase," *The News*, April 18, 2020, https://www.thenews.com.pk/print/646072-corona-cases-in-pakistan-witness-sharp-increase

34. "Pakistanis gather for Friday prayers defying coronavirus advisory," *Al Jazeera*, April 17, 2020, https://www.aljazeera.com/news/2020/04/pakistanis-gather-friday-prayers-defying-coronavirus-advisory-200417104036221.html

35. "Clerics, people flout Friday congregation restrictions," *Dawn*, April 04, 2020, https://www.dawn.com/news/1546276; Also, see "More than 50 clerics warn govt not to further restrictions on prayer congregations," *Dawn*, April 14, 2020, https://www.dawn.com/news/1548934

36. "Govt, ulema reach consensus on conditional prayer congregations during Ramazan," *Express Tribune*, April 18, 2020, https://tribune.com.pk/story/2201078/covid-19-president-alvi-calls-taking-precautionary-measures-mosques-ramazan

37. "Khatme Shifa also known as 'Ayat ash-Shifa' comprised of Six Quranic Verses of Healing." See these verses in Arabic and English here, "Six Quranic Verses of Healing: Ayat Ash-Shifa," Eshaykh, November 27, 2010, https://eshaykh.com/quran-tafsir/ayat-ash-shifa/. (Accessed on August 15, 2020).

38. "25,000 perform 'Khatme Shifa' to fight coronavirus in Lakshmipur," *Dhaka Tribune*, March 18, 2020, https://www.dhakatribune.com/bangladesh/nation/2020/03/18/25000-muslims-perform-khatme-shifa-to-fight-coronavirus-in-lakshmipur

39. "Bangladesh," *Worldometers*, July 18, 2020, https://www.worldometers.info/coronavirus/country/bangladesh/ (Accessed on July 20, 2020).

40. "Like Tablighi Jamaat in India, Sri Lanka's coronavirus fight also threatened by a religious gathering," *India TV News*, April 05, 2020, https://www.indiatvnews.com/news/world/like-tablighi-jamaat-in-india-sri-lanka-s-coronavirus-fight-also-threatened-by-a-religious-gathering-604802

41. WHO, "Practical considerations and recommendations for religious leaders and faith-based communities in the context of COVID-19: Interim guidance," April 07, 2020, https://www.who.int/publications/i/item/practical-considerations-and-recommendations-for-religious-leaders-and-faith-based-communities-in-the-context-of-covid-19

References

Al Jazeera, (March 4, 2020), "Coronavirus is changing the way Muslims worship across the world", Retrieved from, https://www.aljazeera.com/news/2020/03/muslims-advised-stop-coronavirus-spread-200304160256140.html.

Business Today, (June 23, 2020), "Coronavirus pandemic: Religious, leisure gatherings helping COVID-19 spread in many countries, says WHO", Retrieved from, https://www.businesstoday.in/current/world/coronavirus-pandemic-religious-leisure-gatherings-helping-covid-19-spread-in-many-countries-says-who/story/407719.html.

Campo, Juan E, (2009), *Encyclopedia of Islam*, Facts on File, Inc., New York.

Centre for evidence-based medicine, 2020. Retrieved from: https://www.cebm.net/wp-content/uploads/2020/03/Mass-gatherings-and-sporting-events-during-a-pandemic_PDF-template-4.pdf.

Hays, JN, (2005), *Epidemics and Pandemics: Their Impacts on Human History*. ABC-CLIO Press, Oxford.

Mandaville, Peter, et al., (2009), *Transnational Islam in South and Southeast Asia: Movements, Networks, and Conflict Dynamics*, National Bureau of Asian Research, Seattle.

McCloskey B, Zumla A, Ippolito G, et al., (2020), Mass gathering events and reducing further global spread of COVID-19: A political and public health dilemma. *Lancet.* 395(10230):1096–1099. doi:10.1016/S0140-6736(20)30681-4

Mobarak, Mushfiq, (July 29, 2020), Changes in religious gatherings & practices to curb COVID-19. *Policy Insight*, Retrieved from, https://yrise.yale.edu/wp-content/uploads/2020/08/Religious-Gatherings-Policy-Insight-Final-002.pdf.

Mubarak N, Zin CS, (2020), Religious tourism and mass religious gatherings – The potential link in the spread of COVID-19: Current perspective and future implications. *Travel Medicine and Infectious Disease*. doi: 10.1016/j.tmaid.2020.101786.

Nunan, D, Brassey, J, (March 20, 2020) "What is the evidence for mass gatherings during global pandemics? A rapid summary of best-available evidence", Oxford COVID-19 Evidence Service, https://www.cebm.net/wp-content/uploads/2020/03/Mass-gatherings-and-sporting-events-during-a-pandemic_PDF-template-4.pdf.

Polu, SL, (2012), *Infectious Disease in India, 1892–1940: Policy-Making and the Perception of Risk*, Palgrave Macmillan: Hampshire.

World Health Organization, (2015), Public health for mass gatherings: key considerations, Philippines.

Quadri, Sayed A., (2020), COVID-19 and religious congregations: Implications for spread of novel pathogens. *International Journal of Infectious Diseases*. 96:219–221. https://doi.org/10.1016/j.ijid.2020.05.007

Reuters, (April 13, 2020), "'God is with us': Many Muslims in Pakistan flout the coronavirus ban in mosques", Retrieved from https://www.reuters.com/article/us-health-coronavirus-pakistan-congregat/god-is-with-us-many-muslims-in-pakistan-flout-the-coronavirus-ban-in-mosques-idUSKCN21V0T4

Sikand, Yoginder, (2002), *The Origins and Development of the Tablighi Jama'at (1920–2000): A Cross-country Comparative Study*, Leiden: Orient BlackSwan.

Vyborny, K, Junaid, SU, Khan, LR, (April 24, 2020), "Engaging with mosque imams for effective responses to COVID-19", Retrieved from, https://www.theigc.org/blog/engaging-with-mosque-imams-for-effective-responses-to-covid-19/

Wall Street Journal, (March 18, 2020), "Coronavirus is spreading at religious gatherings, ricocheting across nations", Accessed on July 20, 2020, https://www.wsj.com/articles/coronavirus-is-spreading-at-religious-gatherings-ricocheting-across-nations-11584548174

Wildman, Wesley J. et al., (2020), Religion and the COVID-19 pandemic, *Religion, Brain & Behavior*. 10(2):115–117. doi:10.1080/2153599X.2020.1749339

8 Implications of the COVID-19 global health pandemic on ASEAN's security community

Rusdi Omar and Knocks Tapiwa Zengeni

Introduction

The increasing salience of non-traditional security issues such as the spread of infectious diseases warrants a new take on the multilateral cooperative security approach in South East Asia. South East Asia, through several regional frameworks such as the Association of South Asian Nations (ASEAN), the ASEAN Regional Forum (ARF), the ASEAN Security Community (ASC), and ASEAN Plus three, has so far been a successful case for regional cooperation. At a broader level, forums like the Asia-Pacific Economic Cooperation (APEC) and the East Asia Summit (EAS) have brought East Asian states together around issues affecting the region. As a matter of fact, in our chapter, the emphasis will be on ASEAN, which remains the most important institutional framework for security cooperation in East Asia. What is already evident is that regional integration is most pronounced in East Asia outside Europe (Buszynski, 1997/98; Narine, 1998; Patrick, 2013). Ideally, the emergence of strong regional and sub-regional organizations in South East Asia is a positive development because it may provide more effective channels for addressing transnational problems. After all, member states of such regional bodies may confront similar threats, possess closer cultural ties, and have longer memories of cooperation. In the dominant literature, thus, ASEAN is often presented as a model of an emerging security community in international Affairs (Acharya, 1991; Chau, 2008). It is notable that ASEAN's emerging security community is heavily dependent on its normative process of consensus building and respect for the principle of state sovereignty in managing security threats. It is worth reflecting though that despite the emergence of the ASEAN "security community" the institution has been castigated for its inability to resolve conflicts and challenges (Chau, 2008). Some of the notable conflicts and crises include the Asian financial crisis of 1997, the persistent haze pollution emanating from the regional powerhouse of Indonesia, and the East Timor crisis of 1999. Furthermore, recent developments in South East Asia in the post-Cold War era such as the ASEAN's expansion as well as the establishment of complementary bodies such as Asia Regional Forum (ARF), ASEAN Plus three, Asia-Pacific Economic Cooperation (APEC), and East Asia Summit (EAS) has diluted ASEAN's cohesion as well accentuating

DOI: 10.4324/9781003197416-8

redundancy. Consequently, some scholars dismiss the notion of ASEAN's nascent security community by highlighting the inherent institutional weaknesses (Leifer, 1999). These skeptics and doubters assert that ASEAN continues to be underpinned by an intergovernmental process of cooperation.

Notably, the substance of world politics has changed in recent years, which may require new approaches to the management of global and regional security. The world may be approaching a tipping point due to global public health crises. Global health pandemics pose perhaps the greatest threat to world security in the 21st century. Over the past two decades, the world has faced outbreaks of avian influenza (H5N1), "swine flu" (H1N1), Severe Acute Respiratory Syndrome (SARS), as well as Middle East Respiratory Syndrome (MERS). One of the most dramatic events that have elicited a pervasive, profound, and lasting fear among members of the international community is the COVID-19 global health crisis. The emergence of the COVID-19 global pandemic demonstrates that the key national security challenges of the 21st century are likely to be global and transnational in nature. With this in mind, this new threat environment poses essentially different strategic challenges to the world including South East Asia. The fundamental question for the future of global security is whether today's regional and global frameworks of cooperation can provide incentives for cooperative problem-solving to mitigate mutual vulnerabilities. Hence, the main purpose of this chapter is to examine why enhanced inter-state cooperation is critical in addressing non-traditional security challenges in South East Asia. The second is to show how the cooperation and interdependence among ASEAN member states, as a function of a shared set of values and interests, informs regional policies and leads to the emergence of new regional approaches to emerging threats in a changing world order.

The pervasiveness and inter-connectedness of communicable diseases create cross-cutting challenges for regional security policy. ASEAN countries' fragmented response to the COVID-19 phenomenon highlighted the bloc's ineffectiveness in promoting regional solidarity. Nevertheless, the inherently transnational nature of the current threat of communicable disease provides a strong impetus for regional cooperation and collaboration. The tragedy of the COVID-19 pandemic has made policymakers in ASEAN able to recognize that health security necessitates a comprehensive regional security architecture to protect the region from external shocks such as COVID-19. But so far, the development of a robust regional security framework encompassing health security has proven to be a daunting task. ASEAN measures for prevention and information sharing in health security are insubstantial. There must be a shift in ASEAN's crisis response paradigm to health pandemics, from a reactive posture to more robust preventive and protection strategies.

This chapter proposes that the ASEAN and its member states should work together to reinforce national healthcare systems and contain the spread of future communicable viruses. At the same time, the ASEAN and its member states should develop resilience and governance strategies that may mitigate the socioeconomic impact of global health pandemics and epidemics. The ASEAN's response to global health pandemics should thus focus on key priorities such as limiting the spread of the diseases, ensuring the provision of medical equipment, promoting research for treatments and vaccines, and providing a supportive environment supporting jobs, businesses, and the economies of member states. The essence of our argument is that regional cooperation in non-traditional security in ASEAN should be deepened. But now, there is a much more basic question about whether regional blocs can protect the citizens of their member states from pandemics. Through consensus, contingency planning, and coordination, the ASEAN regional bloc can provide a unity of effort to advance cooperative security. This more effective, efficient, and supporting environment is a foundational step necessary to create a more resilient region better able to address the challenges of global pandemics of the present and into our future. This chapter will thus interrogate ASEAN's cooperative security in the context of regional, sub-regional, and national policy strategies to address a transnational threat of communicable diseases. To be more specific, our objective is to understand how ASEAN-centered regionalism may evolve in the post-COVID-19 era, as it addresses emerging threats of the 21st century. In other words, has the COVID-19 global health crisis provided stimulus for institutional development in ASEAN?

The emerging new threat environment

As mentioned earlier, beyond Europe, ASEAN has emerged as the most successful model of regionalism since its formation in 1967 as an outpost of the non-Communist part of South East Asia (Buszynski, 1997/98). Essentially, communism was a common threat that galvanized ASEAN and strengthened its diplomatic cohesion. As a result, the organization developed features that were associated with successful regionalism, particularly a consensus decision-making mechanism that compelled member states to give priority to the collective interest over the individual interests of member states. However, this diplomatic cohesion enjoyed by ASEAN was degraded in the aftermath of the end of the Cold War due to a number of factors including the expansion of the organization's membership and the formation of broader regional blocs like the Asia-Pacific common security dialogue. The specific challenges that arose from the organization's expansion from a cohesive community of six states to a bigger bloc of ten states can be appreciated since the grouping can no longer be expected to build consensus given the diverse historical experiences and foreign policy inclinations. Furthermore, since its formation, the main purpose of ASEAN has been to "prevent, manage and resolve conflicts in the region" (Acharya, 1991, p. 159). This concept of regional order has been premised on the idea of a security community which entails a group of member states who share dependable expectations of peaceful change excluding the use of force or intervention (Acharya, 1991; Chau, 2008)). Nonetheless, today ASEAN confronts new challenges that will continue to test its diplomatic cohesion in other respects, and which may demand changes in the way South East Asian regionalism accounts for the emerging invisible threats. Perhaps the emergence of transnational threats like COVID-19 may provide a new impetus that may galvanize ASEAN and strengthen its cohesion. The jury is still out on whether this will come to fruition.

Since the 1990s, the world community has begun to recognize the national security implications of communicable diseases. In 1999, the UN Security Council declared HIV/AIDS a national security threat, especially to sub-Saharan African nations. Subsequent international meetings in the aftermath of SARS, MERS, and Ebola have highlighted current concerns about infectious diseases as a critical component of debates about national security. For one thing, globalization has transformed the world scene. With increasing interconnectedness between states and increasing travel, health has ceased to be "national" and has become "global." From the movement of countless migrants and refugees to tourists and business travelers on international flights to the regular shipment of goods, the potential for the spread of infectious diseases across the globe has never been greater. In an era of expanding global travel and trade, it is evidently impossible to adequately protect the health of ASEAN member states' populations without addressing infectious diseases in other parts of the world. As a result of our hyper-mobility that is enabled by globalization, distance and national borders have ceased to be important barriers to the movement of infectious agents and viruses.

The COVID-19 global pandemic is one of the major trends likely to shape the security environment in the world including Southeast Asia over the next few years. The COVID-19 phenomenon remains the single most important driver of inter-state dynamics across the globe. It has brought home to all states that they have a vested interest in defeating this global pandemic as the precondition for a resumption of economic growth in their domestic economies. Notably, recovery from the COVID-19 crisis can only be made possible through high-level multilateral cooperation and coordination at global and regional levels coupled with national economic stimulus packages as well as comprehensive national security frameworks. Consequently, a major net result of the COVID-19 global health crisis has been to accelerate the shift from traditional security to non-traditional security. The most dramatic manifestation of this shift has been to reinforce health security as a major element in national security calculus (Curson & McRandle, 2005). In recent years, states are increasingly recognizing the salience of non-traditional security issues as a major factor shaping the security environment (Arase, 2010; Brower & Chalk, 2003; Caballero-Anthony, 2009; Curson & McRandle, 2005; Hameiri, & Jones, 2013; McInnes & Lee, 2006; Raffin, & Brassard, 2014; Teng & Morales, 2013a). Because non-traditional security issues are transnational in nature and beyond the ability of any state to resolve, they are more amenable to multilateral cooperative security approaches.

In the aftermath of COVID-19, it is scarcely surprising, then, that states should give priority to security cooperation to address non-traditional threats. It is debatable whether each and every non-traditional issue should be "securitized" and treated as a threat to national security. Submissions to the Asia Regional Forum's Annual Security Outlook 2009, for instance, identified twelve non-traditional security threats, namely: "terrorism, piracy, transnational crime, small arms and light weapons smuggling, money laundering, drug trafficking, people smuggling, illegal migration, illegal logging, illegal fishing, avian influenza and swine flu, and climate change" (Thayer, 2010, p. 10–11). The extent to which the armed forces, as distinct from law enforcement, customs, immigration, and public health officials, should be involved in addressing non-traditional issues is a matter of debate within individual countries. But it is clear from evolving trends such as COVID-19 that armed forces will be increasingly involved in addressing these security challenges, particularly in responding to large-scale natural disasters, terrorism, and deadly health pandemics. In order to effectively respond to global health pandemics that are occurring in recent years, it is first necessary to understand the link between health pandemics and security. After all, health pandemics affect national and global security (Brower, & Chalk, 2003; Curson & McRandle, 2005; MaClean, 2008; McInnes & Lee, 2006).

In the past century, the primary security discourse has been state-centric, aiming to protect the nation's territorial integrity from an outside military threat. Today, the state-centric security paradigm is too narrow to prevent all external threats to states. As a result, security is too interdependent an issue to be defined purely in military terms and ASEAN member states face a myriad of transnational security threats. Some of the non-traditional threats that require non-traditional responses include climate change, food security, water security, and communicable diseases. Writing in 2007, Williams and Job had a premonition about the COVID-19 phenomenon when they observed that "on the issue of health security, the prospect of a pandemic outbreak of avian influenza, more commonly known as the 'bird flu,' has policymakers and experts alike deeply concerned about a lack of preparedness" (p. 2). A global pandemic such as COVID-19 is a type of insecurity or threat that blurs the traditional notion of national security. An invisible threat that knows no borders makes the response much more complicated to address. What is clear is that military responses and nation-centered politics alone are not capable of delivering solutions to "these threats without a threatener" such as pandemics (Patrick, 2013, p. 31).

The multifaceted nature of 21st Century security threats requires a fresh look at security, which allows countries to be better prepared for contingencies related to health pandemics (Brower & Chalk, 2003; MaClean, 2008). Secure states do not automatically mean secure peoples and communicable diseases are proving that. Just because a nation's territory is secure from outside military attack does not necessarily mean the people within the country are safe from socioeconomic upheaval and other forms of calamities. This has become very clear during the COVID-19 global health pandemic, which broke out in China in 2019. This is just one example of how communicable diseases can create instability within seemingly secure states, which deeply affect the lives of people, food security, and the economy both within South East Asia and globally (Dipankar, 2003). After all, public health is one of the basic elements upon which national security rests. Without a healthy and secure citizenry, free from fear of major health risks, Asian countries cannot prosper, expand their economy, adequately secure their borders and maintain their national and international integrity. In this respect, any government that cannot maintain the health and wellbeing of its citizens is failing in one of its most fundamental responsibilities. Unsurprisingly, the global COVID-19 crisis drove home to many countries their vulnerability to global forces such as the spread of infectious diseases. In this regard, global health crises influence people's everyday lives because by killing many people, they cause prolonged global economic crises. While effective responses to global pandemics allow human societies to flourish, readiness and preparedness failures in responding to health pandemics can negatively impact societies. Various health pandemics fluctuations throughout history caused entire civilizations to suffer and there are numerous instances of pandemics leading to political and socioeconomic upheaval.

The health security domain will continue to grow in importance in the coming years as the world continues to battle and recover from the global COVID-19 pandemic and resume economic activities. This will underscore the strategic importance of non-traditional security concerns. There are positive features of this trend. For instance, all nations in the world will have a vital common interest in maintaining the health security of their people on which their economic prosperity and national security depend. This will be the case especially for the Malaysian economy that depends on vital energy resources and food security. The heightened importance of the health security domain also raises the possibility of increased multilateral cooperation to guarantee national security. As threats become more diverse and transnational, state security interests are no longer independent but shared. As can be seen in the COVID-19 global health crisis, traditional national security is being supplanted by international security. There is a need to develop new frameworks of national security incorporating broader collective security issues (like communicable diseases and climate change) into our national security paradigms (Brower & Chalk, 2003). These security threats may precipitate large-scale disruption that national public health, law enforcement, and emergency response teams cannot contain. Such a scenario has become vivid during the COVID-19 global health pandemic, which broke out in China in 2019. The spread of infectious diseases is a risk to global security because it increases vulnerability in public health, agriculture, energy, and other economic activities. Readiness and preparedness policies including mitigation will increase countries' resiliency. Nevertheless, the traditional tools of security may need to be deployed in response to large disruptions caused by pandemics, as is the case with COVID-19. In an era of great turbulence, combining the traditional notions of security with aspects of collective security allows ASEAN member states at risk of the effects of global pandemics to limit vulnerability and remain flexible for the wide range of contingencies that lie ahead. As the literature reviewed attests, security is not one-dimensional but multi-dimensional (Curson & McRandle, 2005), and thus, health security must be integrated into the national security discourse in order to prepare for the multifaceted threats and risks associated with non-traditional security threats like COVID-19.

In the 21st century, it has become necessary for regional blocs such as ASEAN to incorporate a wider international perspective into regional security policies mechanisms (Williams & Job, 2007). Infectious diseases now move around the world at unprecedented speeds. Nowhere is safe, and international boundaries have lost much of their traditional significance as barriers to imported disease. Nonetheless, it is imperative to note that the internationalization of infectious diseases is not a new phenomenon. Disease has always played a critical role in human history, and the last two centuries, in particular, are full of instances of disease accompanying global migrant flows. What is new is the speed of trade and human movement, along with its range and the pace at which we have modified the biophysical environment (Teng & Morales, 2013c) As can be seen, the hallmarks of globalization such as expanding communications and flows of people and highly integrated financial and trading markets, facilitate events that directly impact our daily lives (Goldstein & Pevehouse, 2013). In many ways, these factors require governments and regional actors to develop even greater levels of international cooperation to control the spread of infections.

In the ASEAN region, as elsewhere, national security has primarily been conceptualized in terms of preserving the integrity of the state, its territorial boundaries, its political institutions, and its relationships with other states. Since the end of the Cold War, however, efforts have been made to broaden and deepen the domain of national security debates to include consideration of non-traditional threats like bio-terrorism, ethnic conflicts, environmental threats, economic threats, and infectious diseases. What is already visible is that regional security mechanisms need to include consideration of infectious disease inside and outside ASEAN, because such a threat impinges on the territorial integrity and viability of the member states. Intrinsic in this is that national security as well as regional security needs to recognize that individual health, wellbeing, and security are all intimately connected to the preservation of the integrity of the state as a viable political, socioeconomic, and territorial entity. A regional bloc's ability to maintain the health, quality of life, and basic freedoms of the citizens of its member states is one of its prime functions. To this end, regional security cooperation in South East Asia needs to concern itself with the medical or health vulnerability of all populations in ASEAN and to provide, as far as possible, a risk-free and secure environment.

Theorizing regional cooperative security among ASEAN states in the COVID-19 era

One of the classical international relations questions is why states join international organizations such as ASEAN. According to the realist school, international organizations are created and financed by great powers in order to spread their ideas and values and solidify their hold on power. However, this premise is generally refuted by proponents of liberal institutionalism who emphasize that international organizations "enhance international cooperation and bolster national and international security" (Morgan, 2013, p. 32). To put it another way, scholars of the liberal tradition have a conviction that international relations can be cooperative rather than conflictual or competitive. Consequently, advocates of liberal institutionalism in particular (Immanuel Kant; Robert Keohane 1989) highlight that individuals as well as states share many interests and thus engage in cooperative behavior, which yields greater mutual benefits. Some of the benefits that may accrue from institutions include the sharing of information, the shaping of collective identity and compliance, the reduction of transaction costs, and the maintenance of collective interest from interdependence. This liberalist school does not refute the realist idea that states have their own interests, but it asserts that individuals and states are self-interested and competitive to a point. As part of liberal framing, individuals and states advance their interests by developing international organizations to manage growing interdependence and allow for collective action, especially where mutual advantage is possible. To put it differently, states are not averse to cooperation. Based on these postulates, how should the threat of the COVID-19 be mitigated? Are the participating states in international organizations such as ASEAN merely interested in using the institutions to advance their parochial interests, as realists would suggest, or does their participation enhance the management of common challenges, promote order, and allow for coordination arrangements, as liberal institutionalism would advocate? The World Health Organization's growing role in dealing with threats of global pandemics and epidemics shows that as cooperation grows, so does every state's stake in it, giving rise to enhanced support for organizations, rules, and regimes.

In the decision-making process leading up to foreign policy behavior, decisions are more often taken in the national capitals than in the headquarters of regional organizations. Although literature and practice highlight the fact that in the majority of cases, national interests rather than any institutional principle served as the basis for states' behavior in international affairs, in some circumstances, states can be cooperative rather than competitive. In the broadest of terms, the emergence of transnational threats such as COVID-19 raises the key question of whether a state should choose a competitive or cooperative strategy. On the one hand, competitive approaches for achieving security are driven by the self-help posture of states, given the anarchical nature of the international system. On the other hand, cooperative approaches for achieving security include using collective action such as alliance mechanisms. Since states are rational and strategic actors, it may be expected that their decisions are well matched to the attainment of their interests, "given the constraints imposed by their capabilities and the uncertainties they face" (Glaser, 2013, p. 14). The threat posed by transnational challenges such as global pandemics means that states might not reject cooperation because of mutual vulnerabilities among allies and adversaries alike. There are no winners and losers in global pandemics because this invisible threat is faceless. Every state is under threat. Hence, the inclination toward cooperation is reinforced by the nature of transnational threats. Because competitive policies can have negative outcomes when confronting "a threat without a threatener," a state needs to consider the benefits of cooperation which may enhance states' abilities to mitigate the effects of transnational threats like infectious diseases. Nonetheless, cooperation is not risk free because some states may cheat or free ride, increasing vulnerabilities to other states. To counter such malfeasance, states may design governance structures providing monitoring arrangements that avail timely information on non-compliance and violations (Morgan, 2013).

The COVID-19 pandemic raises difficult questions about whether ASEAN can adequately protect the citizens of its member states. The pandemic has already killed hundreds of thousands of people in the world, led to an unprecedented global economic crisis and transformed daily life – and in the process raised difficult new questions about regional cooperation or regionalism (Teng & Morales, 2013a). Very often, domestic or nationalist considerations impede the development of robust regional responses to global health pandemics. In fact, despite their strong rhetorical commitment to a regional security strategy in ASEAN forums, member states treat infectious diseases as a domestic issue. In the current COVID-19 crisis, the importance of nation-states and nationalities has gained new prominence in the eyes of the public. The result is a lack of integrated coordination in responding to the challenges posed by the global pandemic. Each country has tried to bring its own citizens home. Yet nationalism is not a viable solution to a shared challenge such as a global health pandemic. Even if national borders have been raised reflexively and states are now ruled by emergency decrees, a new rise of corona virus-inspired nationalism will not solve the problems at hand. National, regional and ASEAN crisis measures must complement each other in order to be fully effective and achieve the desired results. After all, the promotion of ASEAN awareness and solidarity are indispensable elements for deeper cooperation in the future (Teng & Morales, 2013b). Given that the contemporary threat of infectious diseases within ASEAN is transnational in nature, it cannot be mitigated by any single state; hence a regional crisis contingency strategy is therefore necessary. The ASEAN and its members will need to revise their crisis contingency planning. ASEAN needs to do better when it comes to quickly and effectively coordinating individual national measures when a crisis hits like COVID-19. Negative secondary effects, such as national export bans of medical equipment, restrictions on entry for health and nursing staff or an interruption of cross-border trade in goods, must be avoided, while cross-border medical cooperation needs to be improved. ASEAN stands out as the obvious platform for the development of such a collective response since the ASEAN Charter promotes "collective responsibility in enhancing regional peace, security and prosperity." During the emergence of the COVID-19 global health crisis, ASEAN countries' response initiatives lacked a coordinated approach. The uncoordinated response to the COVID-19 unprecedented health crisis among ASEAN member states has highlighted the ineffectiveness of the regional bloc in providing substance to the principle of solidarity between member states. States continue to prioritize respect for state sovereignty at the expense of their regional community interest.

The current COVID-19 crisis makes clear why a coordinated regional response policy is in fact preferable to a uniform policy. After all, member states' responses to the same crisis vary greatly because the outbreak is different in each country (the degree of infection, hospital capacity, and so forth). From these differences, we can conclude that a uniform ASEAN solution is neither legally feasible nor objectively desirable. But this does not mean that ASEAN should not develop a common regional crisis contingency strategy. The transnational nature of the COVID-19 threat confronting the globe underscores the need for more robust multilateral cooperation due to mutual vulnerabilities. ASEAN Member states did not step up efforts to support each other as well as sharing resources to fight the spread of the virus. So far, the ASEAN has relied on the goodwill of its member states to give support and coordinate the different measures adopted. However, the current crisis makes clear that cross-border health matters such as infectious diseases, the exchange of patients, or joint procurement of medical devices – call for new ASEAN responsibilities and action.

Another instructive theoretical perspective utilized in this chapter to explain the nature of security cooperation emerging in ASEAN is that of a security community. This theory, which was developed by Karl Deutsch and refined by Emmanuel Adler and Michael Barnett, conceptualized security community as evolutionary in three stages. The first stage, or nascent form, is characterized by the establishment of relationships among member states with the explicit aim of enhancing their own national security. In the ascendant stage, ties deepen through institutions and organizations, thereby engendering trust. We may argue that ASEAN has reached this stage because a number of ASEAN-centered organizations have been created to bolster and deepen regional cooperation. These institutions include the ASEAN Regional Forum (ARF), ASEAN Security Community (ASC), ASEAN Plus Three, the Asia-Pacific Economic Cooperation (APEC), and the East Asia Summit (EAS). The third and final phase, namely the mature stage, is attained when "regional actors come to share an identity and can entertain dependable expectations of peaceful change" (Chau, 2008, p. 628). What does this analysis of the security community theory suggest about the challenges and opportunities for a cooperative security framework to build momentum for confronting emerging transnational threats like COVID-19? Drawing from the security community's theoretical premise, institutions, their values, and a shared understanding are key to the realization of a successful security community.

A related point is that the emergence of COVID-19 may re-energize the ASEAN's cohesion by drawing the member states closer as they identify a common threat to regional security, requiring a collective response. Alexander Wendt, as cited by Chow (2005), argues that "a unifying factor in generating a collective identity among states is the designation of a common 'other,' which can be a concrete threat, such as a particular country, or an abstract threat, such as nuclear war" (p. 308). Put another way, the COVID-19 phenomenon is the potential unifying factor that may galvanize ASEAN and strengthen its cohesion. As noted by Buszynski (1997/8), the maintenance of the collective interest in the face of the threat posed by the common threat of communism during the Cold War era was a massive success for ASEAN, which enhanced its diplomatic cohesion accordingly. As can be seen, states generate processes of interdependence premised on common and collective interests. In fact, the ASEAN is only as strong as its members want it to be. Difficult times can teach us many lessons and some of them may already be visible. Only time will tell.

The search for institutional innovations to mitigate transnational threats in South East Asia

Since the advent of HIV/AIDS as well as SARS and MERS, health issues and concerns have slowly emerged on the foreign and security policy agenda of the international community, although they have not supplanted more traditional concerns. However, the emergence of the COVID-19 global pandemic is destined to change the current perspectives on non-traditional security challenges, especially the threat posed by infectious diseases. What is already clear is the need to move health concerns beyond the social policy and development agenda into the realms of foreign and security policy planning. One of the greatest direct and indirect threats to global security remains infectious or communicable diseases. The contention that the spread of infectious disease directly threatens global security rests on the basic suggestion that such diseases threaten the health, wellbeing, and quality of life of all people in the world. The indirect danger arises when infectious diseases help to undermine the social and economic fabric of states as they interact in many activities across the globe. Infectious diseases remain a key threat to human life and good health across most of humanity. Yet, global pandemics are not a new phenomenon.

Throughout history, infectious diseases have claimed the lives of billions of people. The unfolding and staggering human tragedy wrought by the novel coronavirus or COVID-19 is one reason why infectious diseases, long the concern solely of public health authorities, should become a more pressing concern of national governments and statesmen and women. As demonstrated by the COVID-19 global pandemic, the spread of infectious diseases can undermine the normal functioning of any state, sapping public confidence, tapping into deep-seated fears about contagion, and creating widespread fear, panic, and hysteria. In other words, infectious diseases can undermine the economic and commercial viability of nation-states by placing extraordinary demands on the healthcare system, sapping business confidence, reducing the productive labor force (unemployment), and destroying individual livelihoods. HIV/AIDS, H1NI, SARS, MERS, and now COVID-19 demonstrate just how vulnerable economies across the globe are to major disease outbreaks. For example, SARS is estimated to have cost the world economy somewhere between US$30 and US$50 billion (Curson & McRandle, 2005). Another instructive example is the 10% fall in global stock markets, since it became clear that COVID-19 would not be limited to China (Butler, 2020). Estimates predict that the virus will result in almost 3.5 trillion dollars in lost global economic output in 2020

(Duffin, 2020). Furthermore, an infectious disease can highlight and deepen inequalities and vulnerabilities within societies in South East Asia, accentuating existing socioeconomic disparities. Notably, the spread of infectious diseases can lead to regional instability by weakening already vulnerable states. It can also lead to interstate or national–regional antagonisms, resulting in disagreements and acrimonious debates about responsibilities for quarantine and preparedness and reactive measures.

Central to understanding emerging health security risks is the interconnected but by no means integrated world in which we live. The COVID-19 global pandemic underpinned by globalization is bound to change our threat perceptions, our economic wellbeing, and our vulnerability to external shocks. The impact of the COVID-19 pandemic and, to a limited extent, that of SARS, MERS, and Ebola have made policymakers around the world realize that health security necessitates a comprehensive national policy or strategy to secure people from external shocks such as the spread of infectious diseases. There is no doubt that the contemporary international order of interconnected states confronts a number of transnational global threats stemming from increased population movements and infectious diseases as well as risks arising from the environment such as climate change. From these pressure points, new transnational risks emerge and are made possible by the speed and facility of an increasingly borderless world. As COVID-19 hit many countries across the world, there was a clear trend of response in many parts of the globe, namely, denial, fumbling, and eventually lockdown (Dewan, Pettersson, & Croker, 2020). In our globalized world, it is surprising that so few lessons were learned from past pandemics and epidemics such as SARS, MERS, and Ebola. However, what is clear in the unfolding drama of the COVID-19 phenomenon is that the success in responding to global pandemics lies in a country's readiness or preparedness, robustness, speed, and central and coordinated commanding system.

As has frequently been pointed out governments should aim for robustness in their health security systems, and policies to achieve this should take a holistic, inclusive approach. At the same time, attaining health security robustness is a task or responsibility that should not be exclusive to the public sector. As a result of the inherent complexity of health security systems, cooperation and collaboration with the private sector and other stakeholders is necessary. There is also a need to review existing security policies to take into consideration the challenges brought about by infectious diseases as well as by other non-traditional security concerns such as climate change, piracy, transnational crime, money laundering, drug trafficking, human trafficking, illegal migration, illegal logging, and illegal fishing. With this in mind, there is a need to develop a comprehensive framework for cooperative security that ensures a coordinated regional response with full collaboration of its citizenry, state actors, private actors, and extra-governmental actors to mitigate the socioeconomic effects of future global pandemic outbreaks.

Although the emergence and reemergence of infectious diseases is a widely debated topic, only a few assessments have considered a discrete security focus that captures the strategic importance of diseases in national security calculus. Most prior studies focus specifically on the sources and epidemiological etiology of particular viral and bacterial strains (Cuberta, Shuster, & Smith, 2020), while much of the security-oriented literature tends to emphasize only one facet of the overall microbial threat: the use of bioagents as offensive or terrorist weapons (Brower & Chalk, 2003; Caballero-Anthony, 2009; MaClean, 2008). If the true dimensions of the challenge posed by infectious and pathogenic organisms are to be appreciated and factored into viable policy responses, it is critical that more comprehensive and inclusive analyses of both disease and security be incorporated into existing approaches and strategies. Only then will policymakers understand the full extent of the threat posed by diseases with which they are currently faced and, just as important, the socioeconomic and political context within which they operate.

The COVID-19 global pandemic is one of the major trends likely to shape the security environment in the world including Southeast Asia over the next few years. The COVID-19 phenomenon remains the single most important driver of inter-state dynamics across the globe. It has brought home to all states that they have a vested interest in defeating this global pandemic as the precondition for a resumption of economic growth in their domestic economies. Notably, recovery from the COVID-19 crisis can only be made possible through high-level multilateral cooperation and coordination at global and regional levels coupled with national economic stimulus packages as well as comprehensive national security frameworks. Consequently, a major net result of the COVID-19 global health crisis has been to accelerate the shift from traditional security to non-traditional security. The most dramatic manifestation of this shift has been to reinforce health security as a major element in national security calculus (Curson & McRandle, 2005).

Preparedness, speed, and coordinated national effort have emerged as key success factors in responding to global pandemics. Nonetheless, few studies have sought to develop models or frameworks on non-traditional security threats that improve countries' readiness and preparedness when facing the spread of infectious diseases at unprecedented levels. This is mainly the result of the sheer complexity of the task since health threats such as pandemics are unpredictable, transient, and transnational. The COVID-19 phenomenon, just like other pandemics, does not fit the conventional traditional security pattern premised on individual state security responsibilities, military security problems, as well as domestic versus external problems. More complicated than that, health pandemics are non-geographical. The Westphalian notion of territorial demarcations of responsibility makes little sense because the spread of infectious diseases knows no boundaries. Primarily focused on traditional security threats such as military attacks, past studies have used state-centric approaches to security to approximate national levels of response to military attacks. Health security in ASEAN requires immediate action to transform several key dynamics in the national security domain that are currently out of sync with contemporary security threats. Undoubtedly, the COVID-19 phenomenon will hasten this process. However, existing literature and government documents related to non-traditional security form a positive foundation for developing a comprehensive framework for national and regional security.

All in all, there is nothing new about health concerns as an international security issue. Health concerns have emerged on the international agenda in recent years. Key to this increased salience is the emergence and spread of infectious diseases such as HIV/AIDS, SARS, and Ebola as well as the risk from bio-terrorism and bio-warfare. Such fears are logical considering that infectious diseases are unpredictable and transnational in nature. More dramatic, however, in terms of global health impact has been the COVID-19 global pandemic. In a couple of months, the spread of the disease is such that World Health Organization estimates up to 8.385 million people are infected and that over 450,000 had died by mid-June 2020. Furthermore, more than 4.5 billion people are under containment or lockdown to slow the pandemic. The scale of the catastrophe has, of course, prompted humanitarian concerns, but global health pandemics have also begun to be considered within a security context, particularly in relation to national, regional, and global stability. After all, preserving national security is a fundamental national interest. While this seismic shift has taken place, health security has not taken a front seat alongside military security, resulting in ad hoc responses to repeated outbreaks of pandemics and epidemics. However, conceptualizing national security priorities in an increasingly globalized and interconnected world is an onerous and complex task. The institutionalization of non-traditional security issues such as the spread of communicable diseases is underappreciated, even though its significance should be apparent to policymakers. Appreciating non-traditional security concerns leads to the realization that it has strategic significance. The COVID-19 global pandemic has demonstrated that contemporary security approaches that place emphasis on military threats and responses are no longer adequate to deal with the range and complexity of contemporary security risks, especially non-traditional security concerns. To continue to muddle through in this manner is not an option. Few would challenge the proposition that the transnational spread of infectious diseases poses a threat to Malaysia's national security insofar as it directly threatens individual health and wellbeing.

Furthermore, the global food system has become more vulnerable to destabilizing factors such as the COVID-19 global pandemic. Food security is now acknowledged to be dependent on "a complex set of factors which interact and collectively influence the availability of food, its supply chains, its affordability, and its utilization" (Teng & Morales, 2013b, p. 1). What is striking is that the threat posed by the COVID-19 pandemic has jeopardized the overall food security situation, not only in East Asia but across the globe. Countries therefore need to have the means to stay robust and resilient so that the disrupting effects of infectious diseases are ameliorated and mitigated. In such a context, regional security should incorporate "broader society" approach: from physicians and pathologists to hospitals; state and regional laboratories; education, agriculture, and immigration personnel from member states. Consequently, there is a need for a comprehensive review of the ASEAN policy on cooperative security as well as the institutional mechanisms. Current policies and practices are inadequate in addressing health concerns associated with global pandemics such as COVID-19. Despite the need for effective response to non-traditional security threats such as the spread of infectious diseases, there is no comprehensive regional framework or model in ASEAN that would best achieve the desired outcomes for future responses to pandemics (WHO, 1999). The key missing component remains an established regional framework that must produce the coordinated effort that is lacking currently except on an ad-hoc basis as when the COVID-19 pandemic arose.

The future

There seems to be a new realization sweeping through the international community, which has compelled some scholars and policymakers to talk more assertively about confronting transnational threats. This reawakening that has been triggered by the COVID-19 global health crisis has an economic and politico-security dimension. Economically, there is the realism that this pandemic has grave economic implications on the global economy. Politically, there is the pragmatic embrace of an inclination toward global and economic cooperation toward confronting global pandemics, which may pose perhaps the greatest threat to global security in the 21st century. In both advanced and developing countries, cooperation in tackling invisible threats such as pandemics always appear more palatable to statesmen and policymakers as mutual vulnerabilities are visible. The ASEAN occupies a key position in the fight against transnational threats in South East Asia. Cooperation among the member states carries the promise of a region-wide coordinated effort to mitigate the effects of transnational threats.

The emergence of the COVID-19 may have produced the unintended consequence of presenting a common threat, like communism in the Cold War, which may galvanize ASEAN and enhance its cohesion. The threat of COVID-19 and other transnational threats like communicable diseases, climate change, and food insecurity are some of the major threats to humanity. Few would dispute that ASEAN will face these major threats, the responses to which will define its future role and function. The state-centric and conventional approaches to security as well as the present governance structures that evolved within ASEAN to cope with various traditional threats are plainly inadequate today when the organization and its members face transnational threats. There is an apparent tension between the forces of globalization and interdependence on the one hand and the persistence of a fairly old regionalism characterized by inward-looking exclusivity, which were nurtured by governments for specific security and economic interests (Buszynski, 1997/8; Friedrichs, 2012). Taking these developments into account, it may be the opportune moment to concretize the setting up of an ASEAN Security Community (ASC) as envisaged at the ASEAN Ninth Summit in Bali in 2003. At the Bali Summit, the political leaders called for the establishment of the ASC by the year 2020. This background is relevant to the discourse on tackling the COVID-19 phenomenon since the ASC plan strives for a regional initiative where intra-state and transnational threats are resolved through dialogue and consensus. Just as significantly, it can be deduced that ASEAN member states have reached the security community's ascendant phase where ties of member states deepen through institutions, in turn giving rise to a sense of trust and bonding (Chau, 2008). This proposition is corroborated by extant literature that represents ASEAN as a model of a nascent security community.

Conclusion

The emergence of new infectious diseases and the re-emergence of old diseases in more virulent forms is transforming the nature of global security. This wave of transnational threats is a particularly significant event as it marks a qualitative change in direction both for national and regional security. It is precisely at this point in time that the ASEAN security "epistemic" community should raise infectious diseases, epidemics, and pandemics from an ordinary policy concern to a security issue. The preceding discussion makes clear that both realist and liberal theories can be merged to develop a more rational approach for addressing the threat posed by invisible challenges such as global pandemics. It also sheds important light on the need to develop new regional approaches to tackle "a threat without threateners." Coping with the daunting challenge of the COVID-19 phenomenon will require reinvigorating multilateral cooperation both at regional and global levels. Drawing on realism, liberalism, and security community, we therefore argue that the threat of the COVID-19 global pandemic and other transnational challenges have the potential to galvanize denser ASEAN security cooperation that may give credence to the notion that ASEAN is a nascent security community. As a result, one of the most predominant themes in this chapter is the observation that the latest euphoria of the COVID-19 phenomenon will galvanize ASEAN and strengthen its regional cohesion. In the emerging COVID-19 era ASEAN appears to capture a new raison d'etre – protection against a mutual and transnational threat. Shared vulnerability explains why ASEAN member states are drawn to non-traditional security cooperation. All things considered, the COVID-19 phenomenon makes clear that in an increasingly interdependent world characterized by mutual vulnerabilities, the challenge for global policymakers including in South East Asia is to develop effective regional and global governance structures to address common and transnational problems at the global level. In navigating this age of calamity, contemporary statesmen and women should ensure that these governance structures incorporate transnational networks and non-state actors in finding common ground amid faceless new threats. After all, the experience of COVID-19 indicates that managing global pandemics is absolutely critical to the long-term health of global security, doubly so in circumstances where traditional global, regional, and national governance structures for dealing with transnational threats are limited.

References

Arase, D. (2010). Non-Traditional Security in China-ASEAN Cooperation: The Institutionalization of Regional Security Cooperation and the Evolution of East Asian Regionalism, *Asian Survey*, Vol. 50, No. 4, pp. 808–833.

Acharya, A. (1991). The Association of South East Asian Nations "Security Community" or "Defiance Community", *Pacific Affairs*, Vol. 64, No. 2, pp. 159–178.

Brower, J. & Chalk, P.(2003).*The Global Threat of New and Reemerging Infectious Diseases*, California: RAND Corporation.

Buszynski, L. (1997/8). ASEAN's new challenges, *Pacific Affairs*, Vol. 70, No. 4, pp. 555–557.

Butler, C. (4 March, 2020), "How to Fight the Economic Fallout from the Coronavirus." Retrievedfromhttps://www.chathamhouse.org/expert/comment/how-fight-economic-fallout-coronavirus

Caballero-Anthony, M. (2009). Non-traditional Security Challenges in East Asia: Pushing the Limits of Functional Cooperation in East Asia. RSIS Monograph No. 15, S. Rajaratnam School of International Studies.

Chau, A. (2008). Security Community and South East Asia: Australia, the US, and ASEAN's Counter-Terror Strategy, *Asian Survey*, Vol. 48, No. 4, pp. 626–649.

Chow, J.T. (2005). ASEAN Counterterrorism Cooperation since 9/11, *Asian Survey*, Vol. 45, No. 2, pp. 302–321.

Cuberta, R.L., Shuster, C.E. & Smith, S. (2020). New Models for a New Disease: Simulating the 2019 Novel Coronavirus, Institute for Defense Analyses, Research Summary NS D-12089, pp. 1–2.

Curson, P. & McRandle, B. (2005). Health Security from Pandemics to Bioterrorism, Australian Strategic Policy Institute, pp. 7–11.

Dewan, A. Pettersson, H. & Croker, N. (April 16, 2020). As Governments Fumbled Their Coronavirus Response, These Four Got It Right. Here's How. *CNN*. Retrieved from https://edition.cnn.com/2020/04/16/world/coronavirus-response-lessons-learned-intl/index.html

Dipankar Banjeree. (2003). Foreword. In Adil Najam (ed), *Environment, Development, and Human Security: Perspectives from South Asia* (i–ii). Lanham, MD: University Press of America.

Duffin, E. (4 June, 2020). "Impact of the Coronavirus Pandemic on the Global Economy – Statistics & Facts." Retrieved from https://www.statista.com/topics/6139/covid-19-impact-on-the-global-economy/

Friedrichs, J. (2012). East Asian Regional Security: What the ASEAN Family can (Not) Do, *Asian Survey*, Vol. 52, No. 4, pp. 754–776.

Glaser, C.L. (2013). Realism. In A. Collins (ed), *Contemporary Security Studies*, 3rd ed., pp. 14–27. Oxford: Oxford University Press.

Goldstein, J.S. & Pevehouse, J.C. (2013). *International Relations*, 10th edn. Boston: Pearson.

Hameiri, S. & Jones, L. (2013). The Politics and Governance of Non-Traditional Security, *International Studies Quarterly*, Vol. 57, No. 3, pp. 462–473.

Keohane, Robert. (1989). *International Institutions And State Power: Essays in International Relation Theory*. London: Routledge.

Leifer, M. (1999). The ASEAN Peace Process: A Category Mistake, *Pacific Review*, Vol. 12, No. 1, pp. 25–38.

MaClean, S.J. (2008). Microbes, Mad Cows and Militaries: Exploring the Links Between Health and Security, *Security Dialogue*, Vol. 39, No. 5, pp. 475–494.

McInnes, C & Lee, K. (2006). Health, Security and Foreign Policy, *Review of International Studies*, Vol. 32, No. 1, pp. 5–23.

Morgan, P. (2013). Liberalism. In A. Collins (ed), *Contemporary Security Studies*, 3rd (pp. 28–41). Oxford: Oxford University Press.

Narine, S. (1998). ASEAN and the Management of Regional Security, *Pacific Affairs*, Vol. 2, pp. 195–214.

Patrick, S. (2013). The Evolving Structure of World Politics, 1991–2011. In G. Lundestad (ed), *International relations since the End of the Cold War* (pp. 16–41). Oxford: Oxford University Press.

Raffin, A. & Brassard, C. (2014). Introduction: In/Security Issues in Contemporary Southeast Asia, *Asian Journal of Social Science*, Vol. 42, No. 1/2, pp. 3–7.

Teng, P. & Morales, M.C.S. (2013a). Food Security Robustness: A Driver of Enhanced Regional Cooperation? *RSIS Policy Brief No. PO13-05*. S. Rajaratnam School of International Studies.

Teng, P. & Morales, M.C.S. (2013b). A New Paradigm for Food Security: Robustness as an End Goal, *NTC Policy Brief No. PO13-05*. S. Rajaratnam School of International Studies.

Teng, P. & Morales, M.C.S. (2013c). "Rethinking Food Security: Robustness as a Paradigm for Stability," RSIS Commentaries No. 111 (Singapore: S. Rajaratnam School of International Studies (RSIS). Retrieved from https://www.rsis.edu.sg/wp-content/uploads/2014/07/PB140331_Food_Security_Robustness.pdf

Thayer, C.A. (2010). Major Trends Shaping the Security Environment, Australian Strategic Policy Institute, pp. 7–12.

Williams, E.E. & Job, B.L. (2007). The Imperative of Multilateral Security. In Brian L. Job and Erin Elizabeth Williams (eds), *CSCAP Regional Security Outlook 2007*. Council for Security Cooperation in the Asia Pacific.

World Health Organization (WHO), (1999). "Report on Infectious Diseases: Removing Obstacles to Healthy Development." Retrieved from http://www.who.org/infectious.disease-report/pages/textonly.html, pp. 1–2.

9 Terrorism and biological weapons

Shane Britten

Introduction

While the ultimate goals of terrorism have differed based on geopolitics, regional agendas, and even personal motivation, one common theme is to create fear. Terrorism is the calculated use of violence to create a general climate of fear in a population and thereby bring about a particular political objective.[1] This means the vector of creating that fear is a tool, most likely selected by the individual terrorist or group of terrorists due to familiarity, a particular predilection, opportunity, or proven success.

Infectious diseases were recognized for their potential impact on people and armies as early as 600 BC.[2] While the diseases and approaches to their use have changed in the last 27 centuries, one consistent factor has been the view of some extremist groups that the disproportionate impact of biological weapons makes them a high priority for purchase, manufacture, and weaponization. This is demonstrated in more modern times by the activities of Aum Shinrikyo in Japan, where on March 18, 1995, members of the group attacked the Tokyo Subway system with sarin gas, a synthetic organophosphorus compound.[3]

More recently, the discovery of a laptop in Syria in 2014 that contained lessons for making bubonic plague bombs and the use of other bioweapons shows active interest in bioterrorism from Islamic State.[4] In 2015, an Islamic State extremist in Paris was found with the makings of a crude animal bomb, indicating further experimentation with biological weapons.[5]

Islamic State and COVID-19

So what does Islamic State, the most prominent extremist group in modern times, think of COVID-19? The answers lie in the group's sophisticated and wide-reaching online presence, where on a variety of platforms and to a broad spectrum of individuals, the group provides guidance on everything from religious matters to targets of interest and training manuals to provide inspiration and skills to would-be "lone-wolf" attackers.

Many supporters and facilitators of the Islamic State's online messaging appeared to initially suggest COVID-19 was divine intervention, with apostate

DOI: 10.4324/9781003197416-9

Governments and people being punished for their lack of belief or conviction. The Islamic State media unit Bunat Alamjad distributed a poster in Arabic through social media channels on March 2, 2020, showing Chinese President Xi Jinping and North Korean Supreme Leader Kim Jong-un and mocking "disbelieving" countries for their lack of progress in containing COVID-19.[6]

On March 19, 2020, a pro-al-Qa'ida group published an article that labeled Sunni Muslim victims of COVID-19 as martyrs. In this narrative, the author regards COVID-19 as a soldier unleashed by God on the sects of disbelief. The author, Khalid al-Saba'i, urged readers to capitalize on the situation and to maintain assaults during the pandemic.[7]

Throughout March 2020, the message from supporters of the Islamic State and aligned groups was similar, expressing joy at the spread of COVID-19. Supporters shared graphics and charts on infection and mortality rates, with users expressing glee and celebrating the range of casualties around the world. The view of these users is most noted in a message stating that COVID-19 was "doing the works of the mujahideen."[8]

Messages were promulgated on a variety of social media platforms, most notably Telegram, calling for followers to declare their faith through action, stating the best protection from the virus was belief in God. Messages included that "no disease can harm even a hair of a believer" and that the United States was being punished for its decadent ways by civil unrest, violence, and the rapid spread of the disease across the continent.

In the Islamic State publication al-Naba, the writer noted that more Americans had died from the virus than all of those in the September 11 attacks, making the virus God's smallest soldier that demonstrated the falsehood in worshipping America.

Although key figures in Islamic State appeared initially hesitant to refer to COVID-19 as a punishment from God, they subsequently embraced that narrative, calling on "lone-wolf" attacks in "Crusader" countries, and stating that the enemy did not show mercy on Muslims in Baghuz, Mosul, or Sirte.[9] Regardless of this hardline ideological stance, however, the group did express concern over the spread of the virus to its fighters, issuing a religious decree on disease prevention as included below.

Countering this, however, is the internal fear of COVID-19 spreading through Islamic State groups, camps, and families. In areas where the Islamic State has a strong physical representation, including the southern parts of the Philippines, areas of Indonesia, Syria, Iraq, and throughout Africa (including groups aligned to Islamic State), there is very limited medical infrastructure, no option for social distancing and no freely available personal protective equipment. An outbreak in these areas would be quick to spread and the death rate is likely to be extreme.

The fear of COVID-19

Fear is clearly an underlying component of the group's messaging about COVID-19. In early 2020, in the group's al-Naba publication, it issued "sharia directives" urging its healthy members to not enter "the land of the epidemic" to avoid becoming infected.[10] Together with the graphic distributed to supporters to provide guidance on dealing with epidemics, there is some indication that Islamic State leadership was concerned about the potential for the virus to rapidly spread through its supporter base (Figure 9.1).

This in itself defines the two-edged sword of biological threats. They are invisible to the eye and poorly understood, as evidenced by both the talk within Islamic State publications of the virus being "smaller than an atom," and the anti-mask rhetoric rife throughout countries with high standards of education and with sophisticated media campaigns designed to reduce the spread of the contagion. In cultures where information is either unavailable, in the case of those with limited internet or media infrastructure, or doubted, in the case of those with vocal minorities using the opportunity to express anti-government and establishment conspiracy theories, the potential for hard to control outbreaks is substantial. To date, these communities have been protected by the global extent of restrictions, limiting international (and national) movement, quarantining those who are ill or have tested positive for the disease, and contact-tracing individuals who may have come in contact with those infected.

In Australia, the state of Victoria is struggling to contain the spread of the virus despite increased severity of control measures.[11] While the virus appeared to be contained across Australia, the recent outbreak of cases has shown how moving too early to reduce restrictions can result in subsequent infections and a rapid spread of individuals testing positive.

In the midst of this dramatic increase in cases comes a range of oppositionist activities by a small number of individuals who are using the situation to spread their own political agenda and message.[12] This includes an increase in the number of viral (a term which seems inappropriate to use in this context!) videos of individuals refusing to wear masks in public, refusing to provide identity documents for contact tracing while traveling, and more. While these activities are not the focus of this chapter, and it would be inappropriate to directly link these individuals to similar motivations that drive extremist groups like Islamic State, in this case, the underlying emotion is fear.

Few things can evoke such fear as an unseen enemy, insidious enough to infect an individual through the air they breathe, with an infection rate far more significant than other similar illnesses. Pair this with a silent incubation period of around two weeks, and the recipe is created for paranoia, social separation, and finger-pointing at sub-sets of society of about who is to blame, who should be held responsible, and who is not upholding their side of the unspoken social contract to slow the spread of the virus.

This fear is not isolated to Western countries or even non-extremist individuals. It is characterized by the communications, relative inactivity, and online engagement of individuals who are broadly affiliated with groups like the Islamic State.

An individual's religious, political, or social beliefs are not discriminating factors for the COVID-19 virus. However, socioeconomic circumstances can play

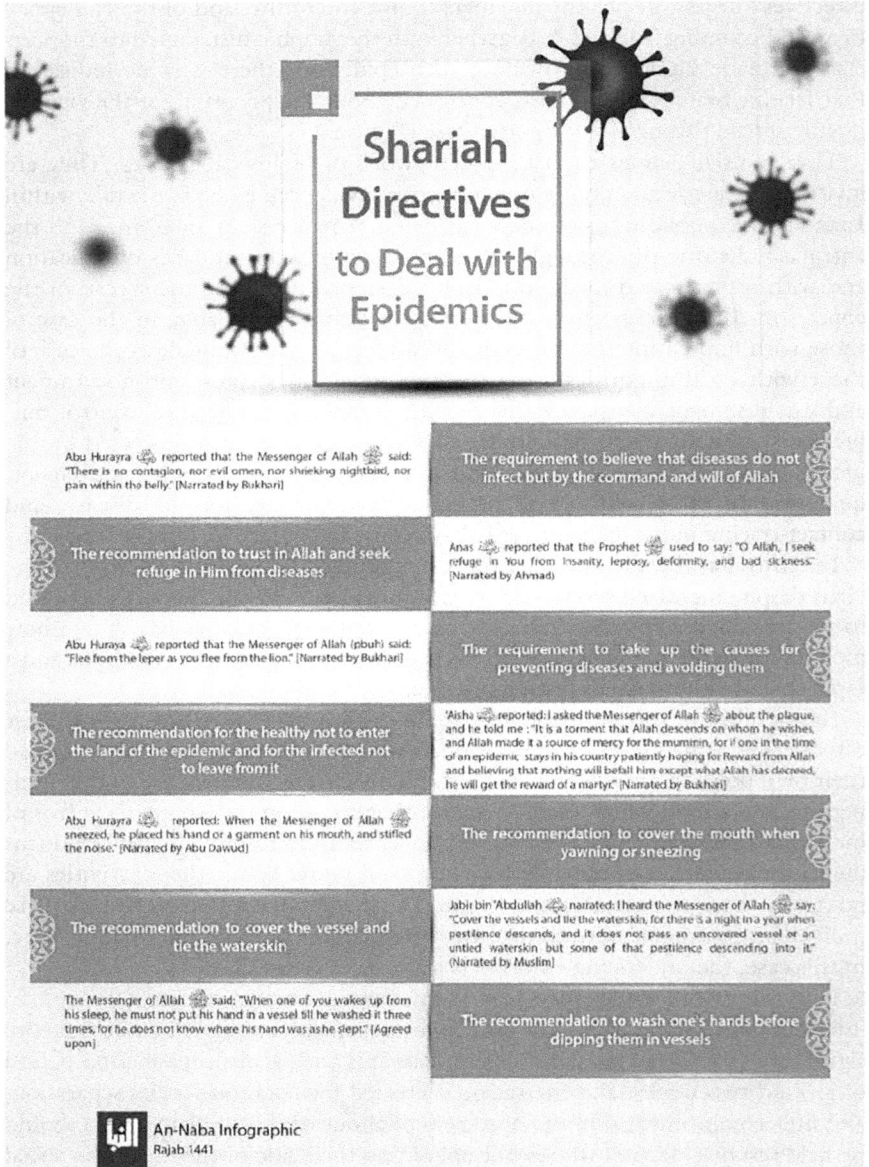

Figure 9.1 Islamic Approach To Deal With Pandemic.

Source: Retrieved from: https://ent.siteintelgroup.com/Statements/amid-coronavirus-pandemic-is-presents-religious-infographic-on-dealing-with-disease.html

a large role in how rapidly the virus can be spread, whether it can be controlled, and its fatality rate. The fear this has generated reflects the increasing divergence between terrorist group leadership and the members or supporters who would be those actively attempting to spread the disease.

The most significant difference between COVID-19 and other biological and chemical weapons either sought or used by terrorist groups is the nascent spread of COVID-19. This is not a biological agent that is grown by an extremist group and targeted to a population, area, or demographic of choice. It is a highly infectious disease that is already spreading rapidly without conscious intervention of the majority of its victims.

The narrative of using COVID-19 as a bioweapon

This changes the narrative of the would-be deliberate extremist transmitter from carefully cultivating a weapon and distributing it to consciously becoming infected and becoming the transmission vehicle personally. This makes the behavior psychologically far more akin to a suicide bomber than a bioterrorist. Perhaps most important in consideration of this is the incubation period of the virus, where an individual may not display symptoms for a period of two weeks or, in some cases, remain completely asymptomatic. This makes it difficult for an extremist to know whether they have contracted the disease, and if they attend government provided screening or testing facilities, a positive test is likely to result in quarantine or similar restrictions or, at the very least, monitoring of their contacts.

Compare this to the laboratory-style manufacture, however rudimentary or basic, of bioweapons and the narrative is very different. The extremist requirement for a *narrative* is thoroughly explored in *The Three Pillars of Radicalisation* (insert book ref), in which the authors discuss the role of personal significance and power in motivating an extremist individual to hurt someone. Comparing this to the individual's desire for prominence, status and ambition raise some clues on why even extreme members of the Islamic State have been, to date, apparently hesitant to consciously spread COVID-19, even if they were physically able.

Conducting a terrorist attack, whether it be by an improvised explosive device, a firearm, a knife or any combination of these, and whether it be survived or an intentional suicide attack, is a public event designed to draw attention, significance, and therefore power to the individual. They may not be consciously motivated by a personal agenda, but by becoming a beacon of attention for their group or cause, they become enormously significant to that narrative in a short span of time.

But consider this in the context of COVID-19, a disease that has killed more than 600,000 individuals, a substantial proportionate of whom are in the United States. Suppose an individual associated with Islamic State consciously becomes infected with the disease with the intention of spreading it and sowing further chaos among their enemy.

The first problem will be deliberately contracting the disease. This means coming into contact with someone who has been tested positive, which is likely to draw both individuals to the attention of health or homeland security authorities of the nation in which they reside. However, this is not an insurmountable challenge.

The next problem would be confirming they have, indeed, contracted the disease. Symptoms may not appear for two weeks, which would mean one of two things:

1 Spending that two weeks in quarantine, without coming into contact with family, friends, fellow supporters etc.; or
2 Attending a testing facility.

There is a chance that even should the individual become infected with the virus, that they are asymptomatic. But should they be tested, they would become subject to whatever restrictions the government of their nation has put into place to deal with the spread of the virus. This will range from different levels of quarantine to stay-at-home orders and so on.

The next problem will be actively spreading the virus. This requires the individual to attend a location presumably populated with individuals they wish to infect. With the world in a mostly locked down state, large social gatherings are rare. An individual breaking social distancing or other health measures, like the wearing of a mask, is likely to be noticed and intercepted early, as indicated by the many videos of similar incidents across the United States and Australia that are spreading across social media.

But the final part of the problem links back to the narrative. How can the individual be sure the virus has been spread to their intended victims? How will they stop themselves from becoming listed as another casualty of COVID-19 without any reference to their political or ideological objectives? How soon before an individual who attempts to become deliberately infected subsequently spreads the disease through their own community, friends, and fellow supports of radicalism, which, as already noted, will be difficult to contain in often low socioeconomic, densely populated areas.

These factors made the conscious spread of COVID-19 a far different proposition from the cultivation, manufacture, and distribution of a more traditional bioweapon. The nature of the disease makes it difficult to spread in other ways, as attempted with the Anthrax attacks in the United States immediately following September 11.

Ultimately, the very nature of the COVID-19 makes it a poor choice of bioweapon. The fear created by a virus that has a long incubation period, high transmissibility, and an ability to be asymptomatic make the vast majority of individuals, from extremists to everyday individuals, scared of the impact this virus is having on our world. While the narrative of extremist groups includes punishing the enemy, COVID-19 does not discriminate by religion, region, or ethnicity. Members of the Islamic State are as likely, and in many cases more so due to endemic socioeconomic factors, to contract the disease as those who are atheists, Christians, Hindus, or any other denomination.

How to identify would-be terrorists seeking to use COVID-19

Examining these same barriers provides us some insight into what steps we would need to take in order to detect, deter, interrupt or disrupt extremists seeking to use the virus as a weapon. The need to "obtain" the virus brings a substantial number of risks with it, especially the requirement to confirm they actually have the disease. The first part of this makes an implicit demand on governments all around the world to track those who have contracted the virus. This means:

1 Ready access to testing facilities with personal protective equipment and testing in a safe, effective manner;
2 Collecting the information on individuals being tested, including their relevant address, travel, location details; and
3 Contact tracing of those individuals to identify how they may have come into contact with the virus.

While these steps are already important from a community health perspective to control the spread of the disease, they will be vital to identify any individuals who may have consciously or repeatedly come into contact with those who have the virus. Most of all, it creates data on the individuals and their locations, which can be used by security services and other agencies to identify trends, patterns, and linkages to individuals already known or suspected due to extremist connections.

This may sound straightforward, but it raises the importance of government agencies sharing data in a way that allows quick analysis, correlation, and cross-checking, something which continues to be difficult within national security communities around the world. Adding health data to this mix makes it one step more difficult due to regulatory and legislative restrictions on how that data is shared.

Some level of monitoring is required to ensure individuals obey their relevant quarantine periods. Given the large numbers of infected individuals around the world, it is not feasible to undertake mass surveillance, but the use of a case-tracking system will allow regular check-ins via FaceTime or something similar, which can be used with social media reviews to ensure an individual is not breaching their quarantine.

Individuals who have tested positive for the virus should be continuously cross-checked for any contact with extremist figures. Together with continual monitoring of online forums and other places where extreme ideas are shared and propagated, this will assist in identifying those who are particularly interested in the virus and how it can be spread.

Perhaps most importantly is the need to ensure our agencies, from military to intelligence and law enforcement, are still able to operate in a COVID-19 safe manner. This includes ensuring they receive training on the virus, personal protective equipment and are able to conduct their jobs remotely or with appropriate social distancing measures. While the virus is debilitating to our economy and society, we cannot let a small group of individuals intent on causing death, mayhem, and fear, to make use of the virus as a bioweapon.

The response to COVID-19

The worldwide restrictions on travel and the economic difficulty of closed businesses appear to have led to a reduction in extremist acts or plans in Western countries.[13] However, attacks continue in Syria, Iraq, and Afghanistan. Simply put, Islamic extremists have not paused their fight in order to work collaboratively to defeat COVID-19. Research of extremist use of social media shows us that groups are interested in whether the virus could be used as a weapon, and it is the nature of the virus, the difficulty of confirming a positive test and the inherent fear of an invisible sickness that remains poorly understood that is preventing its active use as a bioweapon by these groups.

This does not mean we can afford to discount the possibility. While social distancing, business closures, and restricted travel might make individuals come to attention more readily if they breach these conditions, the minor civil unrest in countries like Australia due to tight restrictions and requirements to wear face-masks, can provide a smoke-screen for a well-prepared extremist individual or group to use the virus in an attack.

Government agencies need to be prepared more than ever to cross-reference data sets, collaborate in ways that haven't previously been considered at scale, and introduce new agencies into the broad definition of national security. In only a few months, COVID-19 has become a significant and real threat to the security of many nations, crippling infrastructure, development, health, and economic growth. So while health and biosecurity has not traditionally been "inside the tent" of national security, it is vital that our governments start to broaden this definition.

While barriers will still need to remain in order to rightly protect classified and sensitive methods of information collection and intelligence analysis, the correlation of health data from testing sites and extremist watch lists will be particularly important to identify any indication of an active intent by extremist figures to weaponize the virus.

The consequences of this action make a case for demanding this cooperation immediately. One extremist who actively spreads COVID-19 could infect a wide number of people through community contact. While it is not appropriate to explore in detail the means by which this could occur, one person could result in hundreds or thousands of new cases of COVID-19. While only a small percentage of those cases might be fatal, consider the impact this would have on our society.

Fear is a contagion as much as the virus. The thought of an extremist group actively spreading COVID-19 would create a culture of fear, paranoia, xenophobia and exacerbate already frayed racial and cultural relationships. The fear would grow and spread until people would become suspicious of their neighbors and, much like in the immediate aftermath of September 11, thousands of reports would flood national security hotlines and law enforcement agencies.

Worldwide governments need to use this opportunity to engage the civilian population, passing on clear, unbiased, apolitical messages about ensuring the health and safety of the broader community. This includes vigilance and cooperation with quarantine, social distancing, and other contact-spread-limiting restrictions. This is a time for governments on all sides of politics to provide a unified and unambiguous message to ensure compliance, safety, and limitations on infections, not to score cheap political points or create divides in communities at a time when we need to come together.

When we consider the consequences of ongoing transmission and spread of COVID-19, these actions by governments around the world become important. However, if we factor in the however small possibility of malicious actors want only using the virus as a means of spreading chaos, terror, discontent, and death, then it is vital to curb the spread of this deadly virus as quickly and effectively as possible. That will require cooperation on a scale that is unprecedented in most countries. It requires careful analysis of international situations including what has worked, what has failed, and continued research and development with the hope of a successful vaccine.

The response to bioterrorism

Similar cooperation is vital internationally in the broader field of bioterrorism, and ensuring groups or individuals with an intent to cause fear or death using biological agents are unable to do so. Just because the vector is biological does not change the basics of a counter-terrorism response.

For a threat to manifest, two components need to be present: The intent to carry out an attack, and the capability to do so. Intent has long been something that is difficult to influence and brings in broad issues of socioeconomic circumstances, social disenfranchisement, a retaliatory response, and all the other factors expertly explored in "The Three Pillars of Radicalisation."[14]

Capability, however, is where an effective counter-terrorism response can have more tangible success when it comes to bioterrorism. Capability can be broken into two sub-factors: Knowledge and resources. That is, the knowledge to develop a biological threat and the access to the material or other resources necessary to do so.

Limiting extremist access to resources has been a key counter-terrorism response around the world, from registration of ammonium nitrate purchases in Australia to the ongoing restrictions around other explosive precursor ingredients like acetone and concentrated peroxide. It is apparent that restrictions abound for the deadliest biological agents worldwide, where they are not available for purchase or acquisition.

The difficulty with biological weapons comes from the relatively basic knowledge, and the basic resources needed to create an effective bioweapon. Most of us have been subjected to food poisoning at one time or another, and the bacteria that cause this reaction can be cultivated in a way that makes them more deadly. They can be spread easily. This has already occurred to extremist groups like al-Qa'ida, with field manuals located by US forces in Iraq and other theatres of combat containing references to manufacturing poisons and biological agents using simple methods. These will not be explored or explained in any detail here so as not to inadvertently spread the knowledge.

The unfortunate reality is that it is not difficult to manufacture an unsophisticated but dangerous bioweapon. It is simpler than the creation of an improvised explosive device and far less likely to attract attention during the procurement phase. However, the potential for death is much lower.

These factors make it inherent to our governments to monitor those with the knowledge to create sophisticated biological weaponry and any individual with access to the components of a significant bioweapon. But it also makes a case for the careful monitoring of the behaviors and activities of those suspected of extremist ideals or activities, including continual review of any interest in biological weaponry (or indeed any non-traditional weapon to include chemical, radiological, and nuclear). This information must be shared with other agencies around the world to track the trends and patterns of interest, identifying any substantial peaks of interest or capability development occurring.

Conclusion

We cannot discount the possibility of a group like the Islamic State attempting to use COVID-19 as a weapon. It fits the group's narrative of inflicting God's wrath on unbelievers and creates a culture of fear, uncertainty, and economic damage, all positive outcomes for the group. What it doesn't fit, however, is the individual motivation and personal narrative for many extremists. If the virus is a punishment, why does it not discriminate with who it infects? It changes the extremist from a soldier seeking to carry out an attack to the more extreme end of terrorism and potentially carrying out a suicide attack. But where the structure of radicalization for a suicide bomber is quite well established in Islamic State, it is a different psychological process to convince an individual to conduct an attack using a bioweapon where they are the attack vector.

COVID-19 should have taught us that our governments need to be better at sharing and cross-referencing data between agencies, including those not traditionally inside the national or homeland security apparatus. It is only through this data sharing and correlation that agencies will be able to identify extremist individuals becoming associated with those being tested or confirmed positive and conduct urgent investigations on whether this is a deliberate act with the intent of consciously spreading the virus.

Our agencies must have access to streamlined systems, processes, and tracking of cases to identify their origin and method of contracting the disease. This is difficult at a time when the virus has crippled economies around the world, but without investing in the infrastructure needed to facilitate information exchange and correlation, the impact of the virus is likely to be more severe for a longer period of time.

Notes

1. Jenkins, J. P. Encyclopedia Britannica – *Terrorism*.
2. Eitzen, E. M., Jr, Takafuji, E. T. Historical overview of biological warfare. In: Sidell, F. R., Takafuji, E. T., Franz, D. R., editors. Medical Aspects of Chemical and Biological Warfare. Washington, DC: Office of the Surgeon General, Borden Institute, Walter Reed Army Medical Center, 1997. pp. 415–423.
3. https://www.bbc.com/news/world-asia-35975069
4. Doornbos, H. and Moussa, J. Found: The Islamic State's Terror Laptop of Doom. Foreign Policy, 28 August 2014.
5. McFadyen, Siobhan. Animal bombs are a dangerous step towards ISIS biological warfare, http://www.express.co.uk/news/world/667874/isis-daesh-biological-warfare
6. SITE Intelligence Group. Jihadist Threat Alert, 2 March 2020.
7. SITE Intelligence Group. Jihadist Threat Alert, 19 March 2020.
8. SITE Intelligence Group. Jihadist Threat Alert, March 2020.
9. SITE Intelligence Group. Global Jihadist Response to COVID-19 Pandemic, March 2020.
10. Italiano, L. ISIS Tells its Terrorists Not to Travel to Europe for Jihad – because of Coronavirus. *New York Post*, 15/3/2020 accessed via https://nypost.com/2020/03/15/isis-tells-its-terrorists-not-to-travel-to-europe-for-jihad-because-coronavirus/
11. https://www.abc.net.au/news/2020-07-31/coronavirus-scott-morrison-victoria-economy/12509624
12. https://www.oversixty.com.au/health/body/bunnings-anti-mask-woman-strikes-again, https://www.9news.com.au/national/coronavirus-victoria-outbreak-melbourne-anti-mask-freedom-day-protest-rally-arrests-fines-stage-four-restrictions-lockdown-zone-covid19/e0af41b1-7e4a-47c9-ac12-7d7d48b65c8c, https://www.news.com.au/national/victoria/news/coronavirus-victoria-antimask-protesters-still-plan-on-attending/news-story/044f3103eaf7d72a3fdbb805d31ddbb6
13. Chasdi, Richard J. "Research Note – The New Frontier of Enhanced Terrorism with the United States in Mind." *The International Journal of Intelligence, Security, and Public Affairs*, Vol. 22 No. 2, 119–134, 2020, DOI: 10.1080/23800992.2020.1780075
14. Kruglanksi, B. and Gunaratna. *The Three Pillars of Radicalisation*. Oxford.

References

Chasdi, Richard J. "Research Note – The New Frontier of Enhanced Terrorism with the United States in Mind." *The International Journal of Intelligence, Security, and Public Affairs*, Vol. 22 No. 2, 119–134, 2020, DOI: 10.1080/23800992.2020.1780075

Doornbos, H. and Moussa, J. *Found: The Islamic State's Terror Laptop of Doom*. Foreign Policy, August 28 2014.

Eitzen, E. M., Jr, Takafuji, E. T. Historical overview of biological warfare. In: Sidell, F. R., Takafuji, E. T., Franz, D. R., editors. *Medical Aspects of Chemical and Biological Warfare*. Washington, DC: Office of the Surgeon General, Borden Institute, Walter Reed Army Medical Center, 1997. pp. 415–423.

https://www.abc.net.au/news/2020-07-31/coronavirus-scott-morrison-victoria-economy/12509624

https://www.bbc.com/news/world-asia-35975069

https://www.oversixty.com.au/health/body/bunnings-anti-mask-woman-strikes-again, https://www.9news.com.au/national/coronavirus-victoria-outbreak-melbourne-anti-mask-freedom-day-protest-rally-arrests-fines-stage-four-restrictions-lockdown-zone-covid19/e0af41b1-7e4a-47c9-ac12-7d7d48b65c8c, https://www.news.com.au/national/victoria/news/coronavirus-victoria-antimask-protesters-still-plan-on-attending/news-story/044f3103eaf7d72a3fdbb805d31ddbb6

Italiano, L. (2020). ISIS Tells Its Terrorists Not to Travel to Europe for Jihad – because of Coronavirus. *New York Post*, 15/3/2020 accessed via https://nypost.com/2020/03/15/isis-tells-its-terrorists-not-to-travel-to-europe-for-jihad-because-coronavirus/

Kruglanksi, A. W., Bélanger, J. J., and Gunaratna, R. (2019). *The Three Pillars of Radicalisation*. Oxford: Oxford University Press.

McFadyen, Siobhan. (2004). Animal Bombs Are a Dangerous Step towards ISIS Biological Warfare, http://www.express.co.uk/news/world/667874/isis-daesh-biological-warfare

SITE Intelligence Group. Global Jihadist Response to COVID-19 Pandemic, March 2020.

SITE Intelligence Group. Jihadist Threat Alert, March 19 2020.

SITE Intelligence Group. Jihadist Threat Alert, March 2 2020.

SITE Intelligence Group. Jihadist Threat Alert, March 2020.

10 Enhanced terrorism and the prospect of its use in the United States

An update

Richard J. Chasdi

Introduction

The purpose of this chapter is to expand on the concept of "enhanced terrorism," a condition whereby terrorism is used with enhanced effects in the midst of calamitous chemical, biological, radiological, nuclear, or hazardous waste (CBRN+H) conditions. The framework for discussion involves: description of enhanced terrorism's "proactive" and "ad-hoc" dimensions; heuristically driven extensions of the conceptualization's implications and applications; description about terrorist group splintering or cohesion conditions and trajectories within calamitous conditions.

In previous work, the concept of "enhanced terrorism" is articulated with two of its sub-types positioned at either end of an enhanced terrorism continuum: (1) "proactive" enhanced terrorism; (2) "ad-hoc" enhanced terrorism. In the case of "proactive" enhanced terrorism, terrorist group leaders use traditional terrorism and cyberterrorism to take advantage of calamitous conditions to magnify terrorist assault effects.[1] In the post coronavirus era, what is implicitly understood in the carefully reasoned plans of terrorist chieftains, the hallmark of "proactive" enhanced terrorism, is the potential for enhanced terrorism to have compound ripple effects across the environmental system dimensions with direct and indirect connections (see Figure 10.1).

In comparison, "ad-hoc" enhanced terrorist actions are more spontaneous events, in many cases reactive to political events and institutional processes that occur within a calamitous condition such as the coronavirus pandemic. The ad-hoc enhanced terrorism reflective of the anxiety and abject fear that calamitous conditions create are in many cases directed at ethnic, religious, and racial minority group members who are blamed for that calamitous condition. In the United States, for example, "right-wing" extremist groups have blamed Asians and the American political "left-wing" for coronavirus. One variation of this spurious argument reports that the American political "left-wing" works with American Jews through "5 G" communications networks to spread the virus and achieve worldwide political domination.[2]

In the United States, many of the motivations that drive closer personal affiliations to political movements which promote social equality and economic

DOI: 10.4324/9781003197416-10

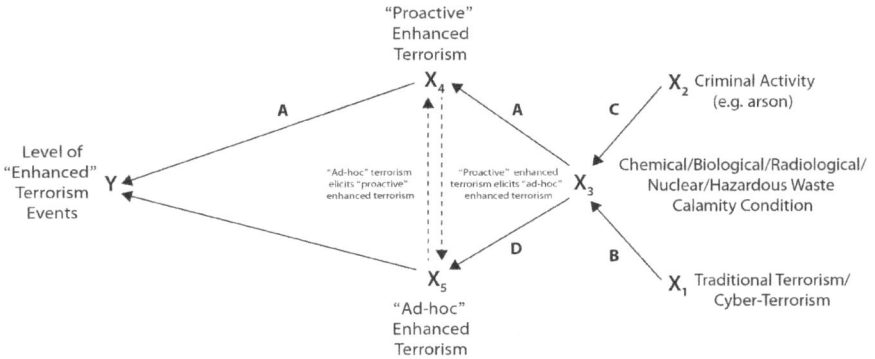

"Proactive"
Enhanced
Terrorism

X_4

X_2 Criminal Activity
(e.g. arson)

A

A

C

Level of
"Enhanced" Y
Terrorism
Events

"Ad-hoc" terrorism
elicits "proactive"
enhanced terrorism

"Proactive" enhanced
terrorism elicits "ad-hoc"
enhanced terrorism

X_3

Chemical/Biological/Radiological/
Nuclear/Hazardous Waste
Calamity Condition

D

B

X_5

X_1 Traditional Terrorism/
Cyber-Terrorism

"Ad-hoc"
Enhanced
Terrorism

Figure 10.1 Dimensions of Enhanced Terrorism.

justice are linked to anger, frustration, and similar sentiments about political, economic, cultural, and social disparities between communities in society. A calamitous condition such as coronavirus works to sharpen those differences; those motivational demands that lead to political movement affiliations, if left unattended by government institutional responses, can increase the potential for terrorism. This resonates with Gurr's notion of "relative deprivation theory," where more plentiful economic and political opportunities associated with one particular ethnic, racial, or religious group, often separated by region, stands in stark relief to the limited economic and political opportunities of other groups, thereby increasing the likelihood of physical conflict.[3]

In the United States, one lesson the coronavirus imparts is that the effects of economic, political, and social inequalities can be exacerbated by a calamitous condition to a point where the provision of basic necessities such as food, adequate personal protective equipment (PPE), and medical insurance become existential matters for people affected by economic blight. Hence, the potential for enhanced terrorism is not necessarily limited to "right-wing" political groups but includes "left-wing" political groups fighting to ensure access to basic food staples and other necessities. Under calamitous conditions, non-violent political movements are vulnerable to the prospect of group fragmentation, where those movements can spawn terrorist group splinter or spinoff groups within the context of inadequate government response to political demands and aspirations.

The role of synergistic relationships in enhanced terrorism

For coding purposes, what qualifies as a discrete enhanced terrorism event includes: (1) terrorism to magnify calamitous condition potential or effects, such as reactions to health security lockdowns or closures associated with COVID-19; (2) terrorism with intent (*mens rea*) to spread the geographical scope and effects of calamitous conditions such as COVID-19, radiation, or uncontrolled hazardous waste materials; (3) terrorism elicited, related, or exacerbated by the secondary effects of calamitous conditions such as anxiety, hatred, or similar sentiments; (4) threats to commit the foregoing in part or whole. In terms of target type, enhanced terrorism, like terrorism in general, can involve a broad array of targets. For example, enhanced terrorism could include terrorist assaults against supply chain infrastructure, where business, as in the case of the coronavirus pandemic, has already experienced economic downturns.[4]

Terrorism happens within the context of bounded operational environments. For definitional purposes, a terrorist system is an operational environment, usually defined by country boundaries or a specific region, either found inside the country under consideration or outside that country where other nation-states comprise a region. Each terrorism system is characterized by a slightly different configuration of explanatory factors linked to terrorist group formation or to terrorist assaults that help comprise the "contextual factors" of each terrorism system.

In a terrorist system, there are a host of synergistic connections associated with enhanced terrorism across different levels of analysis, such as those articulated by the neo-realist "three level analysis" of conflict: the international political system, nation-state, and individual levels, that Waltz calls "third-image," "second-image" and "first-image" respectively.[5] In this neo-realist depiction, explanatory factor effects resonate within and across levels of analysis.

There are also synergistic conditions associated with enhanced terrorism across different stakeholders and enhanced terrorism characteristics. For example, at the stakeholder level, there are synergies between "right-wing" and "left-wing" extremists over the American political landscape that shape the frequency and intensity of violent actions. Hence, individuals and small groups working to preserve the political, economic, and cultural status quo, or perceptions of those notions, might engage primarily in low-level terrorist assaults, in addition, people invested in structural political and economic change to rectify political, legal, and social injustice problems in society.

The Governor Whitmer incident in Michigan is a watershed event that helps signal the arrival of more "proactive" enhanced terrorism in the United States.[6] In October 2020, the FBI announced that a Boogaloo Bois spinoff group called the Wolverine Watchmen planned to kidnap Governor Gretchen Whitmer (D-Michigan) in response to her stringent COVID-19 lockdown measures. One *Washington Post* reports, "one of those charged by the state, Joseph Morrison, allegedly founded the Watchmen group and called himself 'Boogaloo Bunyan' online."[7] That thwarted act showcased the Wolverine Watchmen's extreme version of political and cultural conservatism and support for ideas embraced by the Trump administration. This event is found closer to the "proactive" enhanced terrorism axis on the "proactive-ad-hoc enhanced terrorism" continuum because of the malice aforethought involved; it is coded as an act of "proactive" enhanced terrorism.

Having said that, an upward or downward spiral of "ad-hoc" enhanced terrorism, or "proactive" enhanced terrorism appears to be a function of the interplay between "right-wing" and "left-wing" extremists. Equally important,

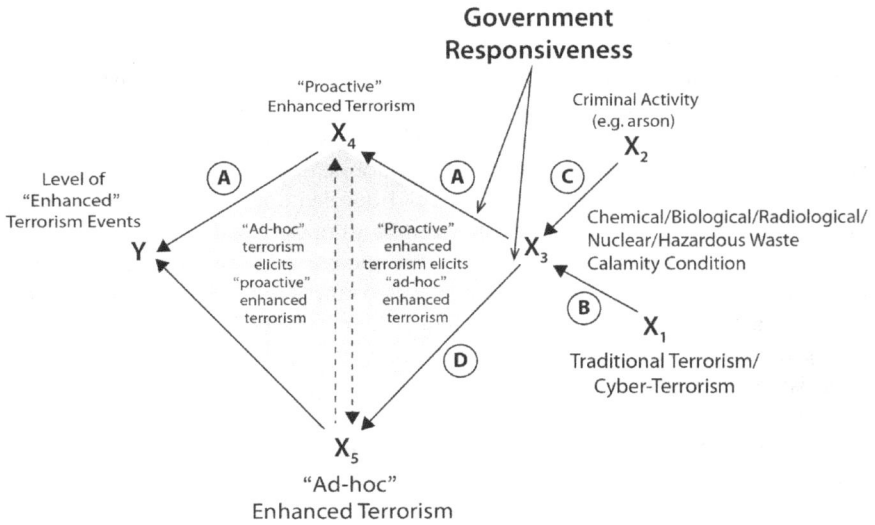

Figure 10.2 Dimensions of Enhanced Terrorism.

enhanced terrorism's "spiral of insecurity," as both Waltz or Jervis might put it, can be increased or decreased by how national government and, although to a lesser degree, how government at the state, province, or department levels, respond to the demands and aspirations of broader segments of society.[8] Both types of "enhanced terrorism" contribute to its overall frequency; in Figure 10.1, enhanced terrorism is depicted as a continuous dependent variable (Y) that either increases or decreases in frequency (see Figure 10.2).

In addition to stakeholders, there are other synergistic relationships to be articulated, both within and between "proactive" enhanced terrorism and "ad-hoc" enhanced terrorism, themselves framed by a calamitous condition such as the coronavirus pandemic. Those relationships are reflected in the two-way arrows found in the two cells of column three found in Figure 10.2. Even though those synergies remain ill-defined and poorly understood, primarily because there is little, if any, empirical data about terrorism practiced in calamitous conditions, it is possible to sketch out broad outlines of possible relationships.

For example, consideration of synergistic relationships across these two types of enhanced terrorism types begs the question of whether or not an act of "proactive" enhanced terrorism would contribute to an increase or decrease in "ad-hoc" enhanced terrorism, or the intensity of actions, and if so, under what conditions. Conversely, it follows the next question is to what degree, if any, does a particular level of "ad-hoc" enhanced terrorism in a specific terrorism system increase or decrease the likelihood of a "proactive" enhanced terrorism occurrence or intensity, and if so, under what conditions.

In addition, other synergistic relationships to examine in the future include the relationship between anonymous and claimed terrorist assaults. Likewise, it remains uncertain how the coronavirus pandemic will affect rates of terrorist assaults with single target or multiple targets, or if targets are attacked simultaneously or sequentially. It is plausible the coronavirus condition will shift those ratios, perhaps with an increase in the frequency or intensity of multiple target attacks in efforts to target "first-responders" en-route to initial attacks, to increase the human contact that is necessary to spread the coronavirus infection.

Furthermore, there is the issue of whether or not the coronavirus condition increases or decreases the possible use of "higher-order" terrorist attacks. On the one hand, an increase in such attacks works to enhance pre-existing COVID-19 conditions not only with the use of the terrorist act itself but conceivably with the introduction of a new pathogen, for instance. On the other hand, a decrease in the likelihood of a "higher order" terrorist assault is possible because such unconventional high-intensity attacks might violate terrorist organization constituent group norms about terrorist group behavior, with deleterious consequences for the terrorist group.[9]

How the prospect of "higher order" terrorism affects the overall ratio and practice of "proactive" and "ad-hoc" enhanced terrorism also remains unknown. Another issue to factor in is that enhanced terrorism works to blur conceptual lines between conventional and "higher order" terrorism. For the perpetrator, enhanced terrorism might have an allure because the argument that the terrorist act was simply carried out in existing conditions appears *prime facie* to indemnify the perpetrator from "biological weapons" charges (see Figure 10.3).

Clearly, these questions become even more complex when the type, scope, and timing of proximate national and state government responses are factored into possible calamitous condition scenarios. What this means is the interplay or synergy of counterterrorism response or public policy response to appease (potential) constituent groups in the mix must be considered. For example, the type and scope of either a preexisting condition of "ad-hoc" enhanced terrorism is taken into account to gauge the likelihood of "proactive" enhanced terrorism or vice versa.

In addition to synergies that bridge "proactive" enhanced terrorism and "ad-hoc" enhanced terrorism, synergies between "enhanced terrorism" and "ad-hoc" terrorism types, and between terrorist assault characteristics such as the relationship between location and intensity of terrorist assault, should be considered. For example, it seems likely the biological calamitous condition that is the coronavirus, might have an effect on terrorist groups targeting carefully planned "proactive" enhanced terrorism. That is the case because conditions where high numbers of people who congregate in highly populated venues, such as sports arenas and outdoor concerts, have been reduced through government shut-downs for the foreseeable future.[10]

As previously mentioned, the coronavirus is so new that empirical data collection and analysis is still in its infancy. Still, it is possible to make some informed conjecture about relationships between location and intensity for enhanced terrorism. For example, one possible effect of greater police presence to enforce health security system codes, protocols, and related matters might be as a

**Levels of Analysis –
Synergies Within and Across Levels**

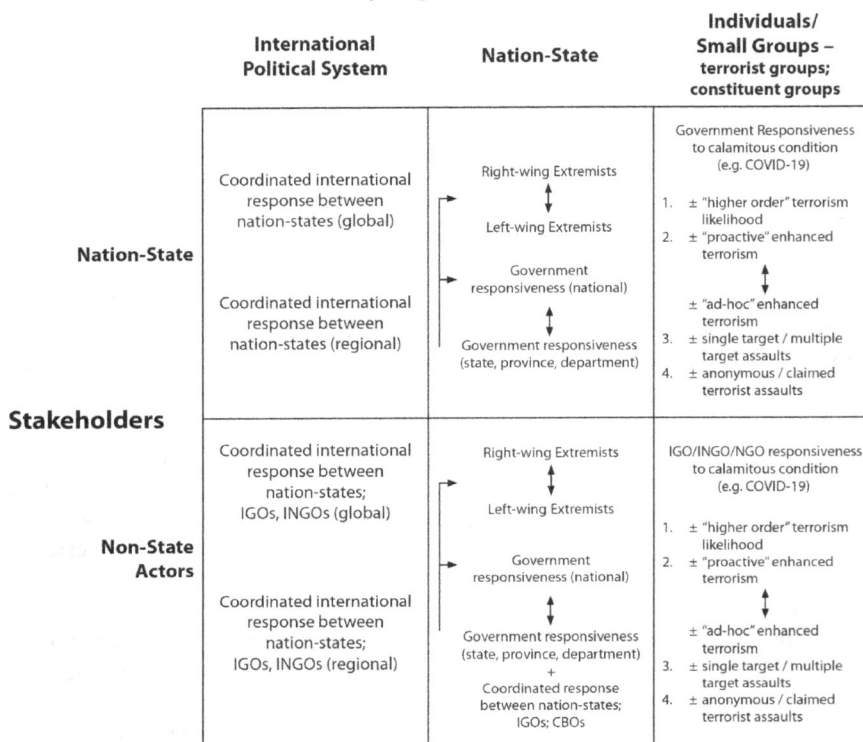

	International Political System	Nation-State	Individuals/ Small Groups – terrorist groups; constituent groups
Nation-State	Coordinated international response between nation-states (global) Coordinated international response between nation-states (regional)	Right-wing Extremists ↕ Left-wing Extremists Government responsiveness (national) ↕ Government responsiveness (state, province, department)	Government Responsiveness to calamitous condition (e.g. COVID-19) 1. ± "higher order" terrorism likelihood 2. ± "proactive" enhanced terrorism ± "ad-hoc" enhanced terrorism 3. ± single target / multiple target assaults 4. ± anonymous / claimed terrorist assaults
Non-State Actors	Coordinated international response between nation-states; IGOs, INGOs (global) Coordinated international response between nation-states; IGOs, INGOs (regional)	Right-wing Extremists ↕ Left-wing Extremists Government responsiveness (national) ↕ Government responsiveness (state, province, department) + Coordinated response between nation-states; IGOs; CBOs	IGO/INGO/NGO responsiveness to calamitous condition (e.g. COVID-19) 1. ± "higher order" terrorism likelihood 2. ± "proactive" enhanced terrorism ± "ad-hoc" enhanced terrorism 3. ± single target / multiple target assaults 4. ± anonymous / claimed terrorist assaults

(Left margin labels: "Stakeholders" spanning both row groups.)

Figure 10.3 Enhanced Terrorism Synergies.

deterrent to terrorist attacks in the first place. Effects of that condition of deterrence might be coupled with the visceral effects on people from government restrictions for large gatherings. All of the foregoing boils down to the matter of "opportunity recognition" and in the narrower sense, if and how COVID-19 conditions will shift the emphasis on terrorist group targets, for instance, or leads to intensification of terrorist attacks as a result of smaller numbers of people at particular venues.

The role of complex systems analysis

The notion of synergies is intrinsic to thinking about the chances of terrorist attacks in particular terrorist systems afflicted with calamitous conditions. The interplay between stakeholders such as terrorist groups and government actors has the potential to create a volatile political landscape ripe for terrorist groups to exploit with proactive terrorism or individuals to exploit primarily with low-level "ad-hoc" enhanced terrorism. That is also the case for lone operatives who often follow the broad contours of political and economic grievances established by terrorist groups and individuals who are moved by political movement agendas.[11]

In my first article on "enhanced terrorism," I mention that organized crime or common criminal activity could also trigger calamitous conditions, such as in the recent case of an arsonist who set fires near the Chernobyl exclusionary zone. Those fires raised radiation levels in surrounding areas to sixteen times the normal rate.[12] That is significant because of the increased coordination and collaboration between terrorist organizations and criminal syndicates in our contemporary world.[13]

Furthermore, the notion that the effects of specific types of organized criminal activities converge to amplify overall effects and public policy problems is a hallmark of what Kaplan suggests are "twenty-first century" problems and what Williams calls "wicked problems." Those "wicked problems" transverse nation-state borders have interactive effects, are poorly understood, are confronted by ineffective institutions or regimes that remain largely underfunded, and are problems that require multilateral actions by states and with non-state actors to confront effectively.[14]

Complex systems analysis captures synergistic relationships in a complex system, where undercurrent flows of ripple effect make the system analogous to a living organism.[15] The goal is not fundamentally to change a complex system but to influence it in some small way to the advantage of government policymakers. In a (complex) terrorist system, there are direct and indirect connections between explanatory factors, stakeholders, and political events known as "stressors."[16] Complex systems analysis makes it possible to scope out connections between explanatory factors, stakeholders, and "stressors," both endogenous and exogenous to the system.

Those direct and indirect connections are, in some cases, characterized by "feedback loops" that highlight potential setback or relapse conditions. For example, President Donald J. Trump's refusal to invoke fully the Defense Production Act (1950) might have constituted a feedback loop reflective of the setback in the policy process stream to reduce the coronavirus infection rate in the United States.[17] It follows that explanatory factors and stakeholder linkages within a complex system have the potential to create calamitous conditions in the first place. Calamitous conditions are the result of explanatory factor effects that converge, while the interaction of stakeholders can inhibit or accelerate calamitous condition effects. Once formed, calamitous conditions have "first," "second," and "third" order effects.

For example, upstream factors to a calamitous ecological condition could include climate change introduced by industrial pollutants with broader "first order" environmental degradation effects such as global warming, soil erosion, and changes in glaciers and other ice formations. In turn, those environmental degradation effects could cause "second order" effects such as drought or flood. In turn, "second order" effects such as drought or flood produce "third order" effects such as starvation, and "fourth order" effects such as ethnic conflict over scarce and finite resources, or migration, or both.

In this case, "third order" effects such as starvation can lead directly to migration or work indirectly as an intervening variable to produce that same result through other "fourth order" effects such as ethnic conflict. Plainly, the full sequence and details of processes and events responsible involve case-by-case analysis and can change with the addition of new indirect connections or intervening variables.

US government support for right-wing extremism – An unanticipated event

Picture a situation where developing world political leaders have "weaponized" migration patterns to settle old scores with the West.[18] The use of proactive enhanced terrorism within a calamitous condition context, either by a terrorist group alone or in conjunction with a nation-state leader, amplifies characteristics, effects, and implications of other related conflict events such as the frequency, intensity, and direction of mass migration. In the process, proactive enhanced terrorism could serve the purposes of both types of stakeholders. However, the calamitous condition that is the coronavirus suggests those processes could also happen in the developed world, where particular communities in society are targeted for political attacks.

The manipulation of calamitous conditions by terrorist groups, and in some cases small groups and individuals on the political fringes, who are associated loosely in some cases with broader political movements or even terrorist groups, was anticipated in previous work. What was unanticipated was the flagrant support of "right-wing" political extremist groups such as the QAnon and the Proud Boys by the government of Western-style liberal democracy. In the 2020 presidential election, President Trump's pursuit of extremist political objectives that dovetailed well with extremist right-wing values, and the tacit support from US Republican party leadership for those stakeholders, was unanticipated. President Trump's now-infamous remarks to the Proud Boys "…to stand back and stand by" in the September 29, 2020, presidential debate made this convergence of right-wing political objectives plain.[19]

It appears those right-wing political movements straddle the line in terms of qualifying as terrorist groups, even though individual terrorist acts have occurred at rallies and demonstrations. While the behavior of "right-wing" extremists largely falls short of the systemic and sustained efforts that are characteristic of terrorist organizations, the evolving political campaign in the calamitous biological condition that is COVID-19 is deeply troubling for many reasons, not the least of which is the prospect that political movements will produce terrorist splinter or spinoff groups.

Terrorism and the United States

The coronavirus pandemic poses challenges and opportunities for counterterrorism planners and policymakers who are concerned with COVID-19's ability to enhance the effects of political, economic, and social differences in society.

The United States has experienced a long and sordid historical legacy with terrorist organizations such as the Ku Klux Klan and other active white supremacist groups. Still, terrorist groups and lone actors acting in the name of real or imagined causes, such as Leon Czolgosz in the case of President McKinley's assassination, and Charles J. Guiteau in the case of President Garfield's assassination, and "spectacular" domestic terrorist events such as the Wall Street bombing (1920), have remained largely confined to the political fringes of American society.

With that in mind, one critical question posed by terrorism analysts has been why systematic and sustained terrorism, similar to the kind that afflicted Europe in the late nineteenth and early 20th centuries, and after the Second World War, has not afflicted the United States in the broader sense. Several factors seem to account for this that include traditional tolerance in parts of Europe such as in France for extra-legal protests, and other cultural and historical differences that either help facilitate or impede terrorist group development, and a critical mass of terrorist constituent group support essential for terrorist groups to grow and thrive.[20]

In previous work, I draw on Diamond's work on "cross-cutting" and "coincidental cleavages" in society and Gordon's notion of "Eth-class" to present an argument that the presence of "cross-cutting cleavages" in the American political landscape with respect to political parties and political institutions, has been a mainstay of a condition where terrorism has not gained widespread traction in the American political system. For Diamond, "cross-cutting cleavage" effects work to promote political stability, by contrast to "coincidental cleavage" effects that produce political instability and social unrest. Seen from a slightly different angle, Gordon's concept of "Eth-class" results from the interface of ethnicity and social class; he suggests that an "eth-class" is self-contained, viable, and politically stable, where political stability is produced by the "…sub-society created by the intersection of the vertical stratifications of ethnicity with the horizontal stratifications of social class."[21]

What both Diamond and Gordon's work suggest is that in "cross-cutting" political systems, where political parties and institutions are broadly reflective of many segments of society, the tastes and preferences, the availability of leisure time (or lack of it), and the values that are associated with socioeconomic status (SES) are critically important. Those factors have more influence on citizen political demands and aspirations at specific socioeconomic levels of society than ethnic, racial, or religious group demands in a political system marked by "coincidental cleavages," where monolithic political demands based on racial, ethnic, and religious affiliation predominate.[22] In political systems characterized by "cross-cutting" political parties and institutions, socioeconomic divisions into the upper class, middle class, and working class, and combinations thereof, have served as a dam with walls to retard terrorist group development, thereby working to contain the effects of frustration and rage, especially pronounced in ethnic, racial, or religious communities where low socioeconomic status "coincides" with such divisions to produce political instability.[23]

What is significant is that in a sustained calamitous condition, those protections in the United States might be on the verge of collapse. The coronavirus has highlighted the degree of political, economic, and social inequality in the United States, and because of the scope of the pandemic, it threatens to overwhelm the stabilizing effects of traditional "cross cutting" political institutions and political parties much like the sections of an ice tray are overwhelmed by a stream of kitchen sink water. What helps to distinguish the United States as particularly vulnerable is the role that American individualism plays in American culture and politics. For many scholars, American individualism is a cultural factor with sources in the Puritan or broader Protestant Christian tradition.

It seems reasonable to assume this breakdown in protections that "cross-cutting" political institutions and parties afford also makes terrorist group formation or splinter group formation from political movements such as Antifa or Black Lives Matter (BLM) a distinct possibility. In turn, that condition, where water overwhelms the dam, increases the likelihood of enhanced terrorism, where its use in a calamitous condition enhances destructive power through ripple effects caused by increased human contact, facilitated by "first responders" and repair workers charged with fixing damaged infrastructure.

Terrorist group splintering and spinoff group potential, and political movements

The cohesion or fragmentation process is critical to terrorist groups and political movements as part of the life-cycle events for each.[24] That process is significant for the government because the capacity to manipulate those processes has the potential to help the government fulfill its national security obligations. It is to the advantage of the government to induce terrorist group splintering or enhance cohesion, if an existing terrorist group or a new fledgling terrorist splinter group is on the cusp of especially bloody terrorist assaults, either to express political discontent or to make a reputation for itself. In the case of political movements, government emphasis is on cohesion enhancement to ensure that non-violent political movements do not splinter or spawn more violence-prone extremist spinoff groups.

For definitional purposes, splinter groups involve direct fragmentation of a parent organization, while spinoff groups involve a more indirect process where for example, factions of preexisting groups or individuals from different factions coalesce to form a new group.[25] As previously mentioned, it appears one of the key determinants to an increase or decrease in a terrorist group and political movement fragmentation in government responsiveness to demands and aspirations from constituent supporters and others basically sympathetic with the cause, who demand political and economic change. At the same time, there are two critical sub-component issues to consider when thinking about effective government responsiveness.

First is what Wilson calls "overcharge," where government, in the face of a multiplicity of demands from different stakeholders, is unable to respond to new stakeholder demands in the political system and the new demands of older, widely recognizable stakeholders with new demands. For example, the US government experienced a condition of "overcharge" in the late 1960s and early 1970s with nearly simultaneous demands from civil rights leaders primarily concerned with political, economic, and social justice issues for African-Americans and Latinos, environmentalists, anti-Vietnam war activists, the contemporary women's rights movement, and the fledgling gay and lesbian civil rights movement.[26]

The second sub-component issue critical to the fragmentation process is the nature and scope of political demands made. Sometimes, political demands and the common understanding of those demands are unclear or inconsistent, and the sources of confusion. For example, in the aftermath of the law enforcement linked murders of George Floyd, Breeona Taylor, Daniel Prude, and Ahmaud Arbery, some activists have called for "defunding the police," that for some, but certainly not all, means efforts to retrain police to inculcate what President Barack Obama calls "stewardship" themes to guide the behaviors of law enforcement. However, for other activists, "defunding the police" means direct and significant cuts into police force budgets.

What that suggests is the importance, especially under calamitous conditions, for government to work with political movement leaders to give legislative shape and conceptual meaning to political demands and thereby provide a chance for new legislation to prevail.[27] It follows that process also involves more rigorous monitor and oversight of the Supreme Court to ensure Supreme Court justices understand their role as jurists who interpret legislation, rather than working to "legislate from the bench."

In regards to the fragmentation process, seven conditions in terrorist systems with the potential to facilitate terrorist group cohesion, splintering, or spinoff formation are described. While those conditions help to account for terrorist group cohesion and fragmentation processes, many are applicable to non-violent political movements with splintering potential. Those terrorist system conditions include (1) number of terrorist groups; (2) number of terrorist groups with shared or similar ideology; (3) number of terrorist group units or cadres; (4) terrorist group dominance; (5) charismatic/transnational leadership; (6) government responsiveness; (7) constituent group support.[28]

In the case of "number of terrorist groups," the central notion is that a higher number of terrorist groups in a terrorist system increases the likelihood of splintering or spinoff group formation, primarily because of wide-ranging differences of opinion about terrorist group policy and scope, and the competition and personal rivalries between many terrorist subordinate leaders, who are potential leaders of new groups. In turn, "high number of terrorist groups with shared of similar ideology" captures the importance of high amounts of constituent group support, itself marked by slightly different political, religious, or social groundings. Hence, potential constituent supporters are available for potential terrorist group leaders to court and recruit.

The third system condition conducive to splintering links a "high number of terrorist group units or cadres" to increased splintering or spinoff group likelihoods. That is the case because of dynamics captured in and described for the first fragmentation condition, namely the high degree of competition, differences of opinion, and personal rivalries found between terrorist group leaders.

The fourth condition, "terrorist group dominance," is a monopoly or duopoly condition where one or two terrorist groups dominate; that also increases terrorist group splintering or spinoff likelihoods because of the individual and small intergroup dynamics associated with personal rivalries, competition, and differences of opinion about direction and scope of terrorist group policy. That dominance condition has relevance to political movements in the United States, where broader "right-wing" and "left-wing" political movements such as QAnon and the Boogaloo Bois, and Black Lives Matter and Antifa, have carved out predominant political niches for themselves.

When thinking about "enhanced terrorism" used by groups with links to domestic politics, and thus leaving out international or state-sponsored terrorist groups from the calculus, it is "government responsiveness" and "constituent group support" that seem to be terrorist system conditions most important to consider. As previously mentioned, "government responsiveness" is an intervening variable between "proactive" enhanced terrorism and "ad-hoc" enhanced terrorism. In that role, "government responsiveness" influences cross-fertilization processes between each enhanced terrorism sub-type. In addition, government responsiveness is critical in the context of its potential role to augment efforts by established political movement leaders to impede splintering or spinoff formation processes with positive inducements.[29]

The role that government responsiveness plays to reduce or enhance constituent group support for both terrorist groups and political movements and compel conformance to at least some government expectations is critical. This is because constituent group support is a lynchpin for terrorist groups and is non-violent that can affect political movement policy direction and potential splintering or spinoff group processes for both.

In addition, two factors play a more direct role in the prospect of enhanced terrorism in two basic ways. Harris reports that norms and values, such as the prohibition against IRA murders in front of family members, have the potential to produce political and economic blow-back effects to influence terrorist group behaviors.[30] If constituent norms and values for specific types of constituent groups with greater sensitivity to conflict limits are challenged or violated outright by terrorists, those actions can affect the use and scope of (enhanced) terrorism.

For example, if the largely uncontrollable and unpredictable effects of enhanced terrorism were to violate norms and "cross the line" by killing children, the use of enhanced terrorism becomes untenable. Conversely, if moral and ethical boundaries are loose or non-existent for constituent groups, then the use of enhanced terrorism becomes more likely. This highlights the importance of research into different types of constituent groups along a spectrum of norm and ethics sensitivities.

Another explanatory factor intrinsic to a consideration of enhanced terrorism use is the geographical and topographical restrictions that influence the desirability and feasibility of enhanced terrorism. Those restrictions work much in the same way that those factors influence the prospect of "higher-order" weapons use that involve biological weapons like anthrax, chemical weapons, or tactical nuclear weapons. Plainly, if constituent group supporters live in close proximity to targeted populations, then the use of enhanced terrorism becomes counter-productive and is off the table as a terrorism instrument. It follows that chemical, biological, radiological, or nuclear calamitous conditions themselves might have effects that constrain terrorism in select circumstances if calamitous conditions are involved.[31]

Public–private partnerships – Enhanced roles for enhanced terrorism protections and government responsiveness

The prospect of enhanced terrorism has important ramifications for the relationship between government and the private sector, namely in the form of public-private partnerships. Public-private partnerships should be enhanced to provide basic PPE to a broad range of communities in society, irrespective of monetary ability to pay. That can be accomplished through a series of tax right-offs, subsidy inducements, or debt restructuring for firms to encourage the production of respirators, high-quality masks, and other protective gear.

In a similar vein, joint public-private partnership programs with an emphasis on teaching computer skills should be systemized and institutionalized. Such programs should focus on teaching, and computer hardware and software provisions to students, not only in the United States but also to students worldwide. It becomes imperative for multinational corporations to assist in efforts to ensure that this generation of students does not become a "lost generation" with respect to educational attainment levels.

In addition to economic resources and political and monetary incentives provided to the private sector by national and state governments, multinational corporation leaders might find such public-private partnership programs geared toward the prevention of terrorism conducted under calamitous conditions attractive. That is the case because such programs enhance the range of corporate security responsibility (CSR) approaches and tactics available to improve the firm's corporate image. Enhanced public-private cooperation in the context of calamitous conditions and the lurking prospect of enhanced terrorism also works to stimulate research and development for possible vaccines and more effective PPE.

A critical strategic component of this process is to manufacture protocol and policy directives that are widely recognized and accepted across public and private sectors. Those should be codified in ways similar to other product standards crafted by the International Organization for Standardization (ISO). That underscores the importance of multilateral efforts and the neo-liberal approach about the role non-state actors play to assist states, wherein this case, nation-states work together with non-state actors such as the ISO, to create industry side standards for PPE.[32]

Final reflections

This essay has described new components of the enhanced terrorism conceptualization that includes synergistic relationships between "proactive" enhanced terrorism and "ad-hoc" enhanced terrorism and between enhanced terrorism subtypes and terrorist assault attributes. One set of synergistic relationships involves environmental dynamics such as the interplay between "right-wing" and "left-wing" political groups or movements as a factor to consider when thinking about the prospect of political movement splintering and the potential use of enhanced terrorism.

Many explanatory factor relationships in enhanced terrorism remain unknown but are articulated in the most general sense to provide the foundations for future empirical work. For example, consideration of other relationships across "proactive" and "ad-hoc" enhanced terrorism begs the question of whether or not "proactive" enhanced terrorism might contribute to an increase or decrease in "ad-hoc" enhanced terrorism, or "ad-hoc" event intensity, and if so, under what conditions. Conversely, this question is to what degree, if any, does a particular level of "ad-hoc" enhanced terrorism increase or decrease the likelihood of "proactive" enhanced terrorism or its intensity, and if so, under what conditions.

Other enhanced terrorism synergistic relationships that await future empirical research when additional acts of enhanced terrorism materialize revolve around how enhanced terrorism or threats of enhanced terrorism might change terrorist group behavioral patterns. For example, the relationships between enhanced terrorism and the frequencies of single or multiple target attacks, the ratio between anonymous and claimed terrorist attacks, and the type of targets involved will require empirical investigation.

One aspect of enhanced terrorism to scope out with empirical data analysis in the future is the role of government responsiveness. Government responsiveness is critical as an intervening variable in two ways: (1) to modulate relationships between "proactive" and "ad-hoc" enhanced terrorism that contribute to overall frequencies of enhanced terrorism events; (2) to modulate the degree of "ad-hoc" terrorism produced in response to government policy shortcomings in specific calamitous conditions, such as the absence of a coherent national policy by the Trump administration to address the coronavirus pandemic in the United States.

The second role for government responsiveness is more functional in terms of its abilities to respond to the particular demands and aspirations of leaders in political movements in danger of splintering or spinoff group formation. In the case of non-violent political movements, a national government's role is to promote cohesion, but if that fails and political movement splintering or spinoff group formation becomes the emergent reality, the government needs to expand its focus to include both cohesion and splintering approaches and tactics when applicable.

Seven terrorist system conditions conducive to terrorist group splintering and spinoff formation are presented to provide the basics of thinking about effective counterterrorism policy that involves the manipulation of terrorist group processes; I extrapolate to include peaceful political movement processes. It is important should traditional protective infrastructure that revolves around what Diamond calls "cross-cutting" political institutions and political parties in place in the United States and other Western-style liberal democracies eventually fail to contain the demands of political groups based on ethnic politics.[33] A worst-case scenario is the horrendous loss of life in a calamitous condition such as the coronavirus pandemic, which includes disproportionate numbers of deaths in ethnic and racial minority communities, that in many cases, are confronted with economic blight. It is no exaggeration to say that would probably lead to a groundswell of unprecedented protest against the American political system that could increase the likelihood of (enhanced) terrorism.

In regards to peaceful political movements, the government might apply what is known about terrorist systems and terrorist groups to ensure that political movement cohesion is maintained through engagement with political movement leaders and effective and sustained government efforts to satisfy political movement constituent group demands. This point underscores that the absence of a coherent, multidimensional, and coordinated American national policy to confront COVID-19 has both direct implications in terms of loss of life and human suffering and indirect implications for political movements with respect to what political dynamics will materialize if such inchoate and desultory policies continue.

Notes

1. Chasdi, Richard J. (2020). "Research Note – The New Frontier of Enhanced Terrorism with the United States in Mind." *The International Journal of Intelligence, Security, and Public Affairs.* 22(2), 119–131 https://DOI:10.1080/23800992.2020.1780075; Gordon, Theodore, and Yair Sharan. (2017). "The Threat of Amplified Terror." Presented at the workshop "Forecasting in the Social Sciences for National Security." National Defense University, Washington, DC, July 26, 1–2, 4–5, 8–9.
2. Anti-Defamation League. (2020, March 26). "White Supremacists Respond to Coronavirus with Violent Plots and On-line Hate." https://www.adl.org/blog/white-supremacists-respond-to-coronavirus-with-violent-plots-and-online-hate; Anti-Defamation League. (n.d.). "ADL Report Exposes Right Wing Terrorism Threat in the U.S." https://www.adl.org/news/press-releases/adl-report-exposes-right-wing-terrorism-threat-in-the-us; Gotev, Georgi. (2020, 5 April). "5G Coronavirus Conspiracy Theory Is Dangerous Fake Nonsense, UK Says." *EurActiv.com.* Retrieved from https://advance-lexis-com.proxy.lib.wayne.edu/api/document?collection=news&id=urn:contentItem:5YKJ-91C1-JCF9-40KV-00000-00&context=1516831; Ackerman, Gary, and Hayley Peterson. (2020). "Research Notes Terrorism and COVID-19: Actual and Potential Impacts." *Perspectives on Terrorism.* 14(3), 61–62, 64–65. https://www.universiteitleiden.nl/binaries/content/assets/customsites/perspectives-on-terrorism/2020/issue-3/ackerman-and-peterson.pdf.

3. Gurr, Ted Robert. (1988). "Some Characteristics of Political Terrorism in the 1960's." In Michael Stohl (Ed.), *The Politics of Terrorism, Revised and Expanded.* Marcel Dekker; Gurr, Ted Robert. (1989). "Political Terrorism: Historical Antecedents and Contemporary Trends." In Ted Robert Gurr (Ed.), *Protest, Rebellion, Reform, Vol. 2 of Violence in America.* Sage Publications; Gurr, Ted Robert, and Barbara Harff. (1984). *Ethnic Conflict in World Politics.* Westview Press; Ross, Jeffrey Ian, and Ted Robert Gurr. (1989). "Why Terrorism Subsides: A Comparative Study of Canada and the United States." *Comparative Politics.* 21(4), 405–426.

4. Pitigala, Nihal. (2021). "The Impact of Trade and Economic Contagion on Developing and Emerging Markets." In Rohan Gunaratna and Mohd Mizan Mohammad Aslam (Eds.), *COVID-19: A Global Security Threat.* Amsterdam University Press.

5. Waltz, Kenneth N. (1959). *Man, the State and War: A Theoretical Analysis.* Columbia University Press. 10–11; Nye, Joseph S., Jr. *Understanding International Conflicts: An Introduction to Theory and History – Second Edition.* HarperCollins College Publishers; Gordon and Sharan. (2017). 4–5.

6. Ackerman and Patterson. (2020). 62, 71 n41, 63, 71 n43. Ackerman and Paterson describe "enhanced terrorism" acts that precede the Whitmer incident that include, but are not limited to (1) train operator Eduardo Moreno's effort to make a train jump track and career into the hospital ship *Mercy* in Los Angeles around April 1, 2020; (2) the call by a "Liberate activist" to murder Governor Michelle Lujan Grisham (D-New Mexico); (3) a call by another "Liberate activist" to detonate a device at the main headquarters of Florida's Orlando Police Department. The carefully reasoned plans by a Boogaloo Bois terrorist spinoff group to kidnap and presumably kill Governor Whitmer, with a similar plan in the works to assault Governor Ralph Northam (D-Virginia), cross a threshold of organized "proactive enhanced terrorism" that in my judgment, sets the Wolverine Watchmen actions apart from other events.

7. Zapotosky, Matt, Devlin Barrett, and Abigail Hauslohner. (2020, October 9). "13 Charged in Plot to Seize Mich. Governor." *The Washington Post.* A-1, A-14; Timberg, Craig, and Isaac Stanley-Becker. (2020, October 9). "Alleged Whitmer Kidnapping Plot Was Foreshadowed on Social Media." *The Washington Post.* A-22; Bellware, Kim, Alex Horton, Devlin Barrett, and Matt Zapotosky. (2020, October 10). "Alleged Leader of Plot to Abduct Gov. Whitmer Had Recent Personal Setbacks." *The Washington Post.* A-6.

8. Waltz, Kenneth N. (1973). "The Meaning of Anarchy." In Robert J. Art and Robert Jervis (Eds.), *International Politics: Anarchy, Force Imperialism.* Little, Brown and Company, 10–20; Jervis, Robert. (1978). "Cooperation Under the Security Dilemma." *World Politics.* 30(2), 167–214.

9. Harris, Rosemary. (1989). "Anthropological Views on 'Violence' in Northern Ireland." In Yonah Alexander and Alan O'Day, (Eds.), *Ireland's Terrorist Trauma.* St. Martin's Press, 89–80, 92, 95, 96; Chasdi, Richard J. (1999). *Serenade of Suffering: A Portrait of Middle East Terrorism, 1968–1993.* Lexington Books, 65–66.

10. Ackerman and Peterson. (2020). 63.

11. Collier, Paul, and Anke Hoeffler. (2000). "Greed and Grievance in Civil War, Policy Research Working Paper No. 2355." World Bank. https://papers.ssrn.com/sol3/papers.cfm?abstract_id=630727.

12. Roth, A. (2020, April 6). "Bad News: Radiation 16 Times Above Normal After Forest Fire Near Chernobyl." *The Guardian.* http://www.the guardian.com/environment/2020/apr/06/bad-news-radiation-spikes-16- times-above-normal-after-forest-fire-near-chernobyl?fbclid=IwAR0TKjvaBPXPV7U5ijU0c3Xc93W9v1zD-BZom5i_HkD4UwkRanTapRiE3UaU; Chasdi. (2020). 120.

13. Makarenko, Tamara. (2004). "The Crime-Terror Continuum: Tracing the Inter-play Between Transnational Organized Crime and Terrorism." *Global Crime.* 6(1), 129–145; Shelley, Louise I. (2013). "Money Laundering into Real-Estate." In Michael Miklaucic and Jacqueline Brewer, (Eds.), *Convergence: Illicit Networks and National Security in an Age of Globalization.* National Defense University Press, 131–146.

14. Kaplan, Robert D. (2000). "The Coming Anarchy." In Patrick O'Meara, How-ard D. Mehlinger, Matthew Krain, and Roxana Ma Newman (Eds.), *Globalization and Challenges of A New Century: A Reader.* Indiana University Press, 34–60; Williams, Phil. (2013). "Lawlessness and Disorder: An Emerging Paradigm for the 21st Century." In Michael Miklaucic and Jacqueline Brewer (Eds.), *Conver-gence: Illicit Networks and National Security in An Age of Globalization.* National Defense University Press, 16–17, 30.

15. Henry, Nicholas. (2013). *Public Administration and Public Affairs Edition No. 12.* Pearson Education, Inc., 67–68.

16. Ronis, Sheila R. (2007). *Timelines into the Future: Strategic Visioning Methods for Government, Business and Other Organizations.* Hamilton Books; Fuerth, Leon, and Evan M.H. Faber. (2012). *Anticipatory Governance Practical Upgrades: Equip-ping the Executive Branch to Cope with Increasing Speed and Complexity of Major Challenges.* National Defense University, Center for Technology & National Secu-rity Policy.

17. Jacobs, Andrew. (2020, September 22). "Despite Claims, Trump Rarely Uses Wartime Law in Battle Against COVID." *New York Times.* Retrieved from https://advance-lexis-com.proxy.lib.wayne.edu/api/document?collection=news&id=urn:contentIt em:60WV-5J01-JBG3-6103-00000-00&context=1516831.

18. Williams. (2013). 16–17.

19. Olorunnipa, Toluse, and Cleve R. Wootson, Jr. (2020, September 30). "President Is Asked but Refuses to Condemn White Supremacists." *The Washington Post.* A-1, A-10.

20. Theen, Rolf H.W., and Frank L. Wilson. (1986). *Comparative Politics an Intro-duction to Six Countries.* Prentice-Hall; Wilson, Frank L. (1990). *European Politics Today: The Democratic Experience.* Prentice-Hall.

21. Diamond, Larry. (1990). "Nigeria: Pluralism, Statism and the Struggle for Democ-racy." In Larry Diamond, Juan L. Linz, and Seymour Martin Lipsit (Eds.), *Politics in Developing Countries: Comparing Experiences with Democracy.* Lynne Rienner; Gordon, Milton, M. (1964). *Assimilation in American Life: The Role of Race Reli-gion and National Origins.* Oxford University Press, 51, 55, 160; Chasdi, Richard J. (2002). *Tapestry of Terror: A Portrait of Middle East Terrorism, 1994–1999.* Lex-ington Books, 50–51, 61 n155, 62 n156; Nef, Jorge. (1978). "Some Thoughts on Contemporary Terrorism: Domestic and International Perspectives." In John Car-son (Ed.), *Terrorism in Theory and Practice: Proceedings of a Colloquium.* Atlantic Council of Canada.

22. Chasdi. (2002). 50–51, 61 n155, 62 n156; Diamond. (1990). Gordon. (1964). 51, 55, 160; Nef (1978).

23. Chasdi. (2002). 50–51, 61 n155, 62 n156; Diamond. (1990).

24. Lasswell, Harold D. (1978). "Terrorism and the Political Process." *Terrorism: An International Journal.* 1(3/4), 255–263. Lasswell, Harold D. (1935). *World Poli-tics and Personal Insecurity.* McGraw Hill, 35, 107, 110, 252–253; Long, David E. (1990). *The Anatomy of Terrorism.* Free Press, 24; Im, Eric Insoon, Jon Cauley, and Todd Sandler. (1987). "Cycles and Substitutions in Terrorist Activities: A Spectral Approach." *Kyklos. 40,* 238–255; Crozier, Brian. (1960). *The Rebels: A Study of Post-War Insurrections.* Martinus Nijhoff, 127; Chasdi, (2002), 2, 229 n6, 29.

25. Chasdi, Richard J. (2018). *Corporate Security Crossroads Responding to Terrorism, Cyberthreats, and Other Hazards in the Global Business Environment.* Praeger, 48.

26. Theen and Wilson. (1986), 19; Wilson. (1990), 10–11. For Wilson, that condition is called "overcharge" or "overheating."
27. Empirical research is needed to determine if what appears to be a spike in US police killings of unarmed African Americans is associated with the onset of the pandemic, generally recognizable as starting in January 2020. This points to the need for data collection and analysis to test specific hypotheses about coronavirus influence on political behavior, including the fragmentation or cohesion of political movements and the prospect of enhanced terrorism.
28. Thaler, David E., Ryan Andrew Brown, Gabriella C. Gonzalez, Blake W. Mobley, Parisa Rashan. (2013). "Improving the U.S. Military's Understanding of Unstable Environments Vulnerable to Violent Extremist Groups Insights from Social Science." RAND Corporation, xii-xvi, 3, 14–17, 22–23, 29–33, 48, 52–53, 71. https://www.rand.org/pubs/research_reports/RR298.html; Chasdi. (2002), 51, 62 n157; Drake, C.J.M. (1998). *Terrorists' Target Selection*. St. Martins; Fleming, Peter A., (1992). "Patterns of Transnational Terrorism in Western Europe, 1968–1997: A Quantitative Perspective." [Unpublished doctoral dissertation]. Purdue University.
29. Baldwin, David A. (1985). *Economic Statecraft*. Princeton University Press; Baldwin, David A. (1971). "The Power of Positive Sanctions," *World Politics*. 24(1).
30. Harris. (1989).
31. Chasdi. (2002), 5; Ackerman and Peterson. (2020), 64.
32. Lawson, Fred. 2016. "International Relations Theory and the Middle East." In Louise Fawcett (Ed.), *International Relations in the Middle East – Fourth Edition*. Oxford University Press, 21, 26–27.
33. Diamond. (1990).

References

Ackerman, Gary, and Hayley Peterson. (2020). "Research Notes Terrorism and COVID-19: Actual and Potential Impacts." *Perspectives on Terrorism*. 14(3), 59–73.

Anti-Defamation League. (2020, March 26). "White Supremacists Respond to Coronavirus with Violent Plots and On-line Hate." https://www.adl.org/blog/white-supremacists-respond-to-coronavirus-with-violent-plots-and-online-hate.

Anti-Defamation League. (n.d.). "ADL Report Exposes Right Wing Terrorism Threat in the U.S." https://www.adl.org/news/press-releases/adl-report-exposes-right-wing-terrorism-threat-in-the-us.

Baldwin, David A. (1971). "The Power of Positive Sanctions." *World Politics*. 24(1), 19–38.

Baldwin, David A. (1985). *Economic Statecraft*. Princeton University Press.

Bellware, Kim, Alex Horton, Devlin Barrett, and Matt Zapotosky. (2020, October 10). "Alleged Leader of Plot to Abduct Gov. Whitmer Had Recent Personal Setbacks." *The Washington Post*. A-6.

Chasdi, Richard J. (1999). *Serenade of Suffering: A Portrait of Middle East Terrorism, 1968–1993*. Lexington Books.

Chasdi, Richard J. (2002). *Tapestry of Terror: A Portrait of Middle East Terrorism, 1994–1999*. Lexington Books.

Chasdi, Richard J. (2018). *Corporate Security Crossroads Responding to Terrorism, Cyberthreats, and Other Hazards in the Global Business Environment*. Praeger.

Chasdi, Richard J. (2020). "Research Note - The New Frontier of Enhanced Terrorism with the United States In Mind." *The International Journal of Intelligence, Security, and Public Affairs*. 22(2), 119–131. https://DOI:10.1080/23800992.2020.1780075.

Collier, Paul, and Anke Hoeffler. (2000). "Greed and Grievance in Civil War, Policy Research Working Paper No. 2355," World Bank. https://papers.ssrn.com/sol3/papers.cfm?abstract_id=630727.

Crozier, Brian. (1960). *The Rebels: A Study of Post-War Insurrections.* Martinus Nijhoff.

Diamond, Larry. (1990). "Nigeria: Pluralism, Statism and the Struggle for Democracy." In Larry Diamond, Juan L. Linz, and Seymour Martin Lipsit (Eds.), *Politics in Developing Countries: Comparing Experiences with Democracy.* Lynne Rienner, 351–409.

Drake, C.J.M. (1998). *Terrorists' Target Selection.* St. Martins.

Fleming, Peter A. (1992). "Patterns of Transnational Terrorism in Western Europe, 1968–1997: A Quantitative Perspective." [Unpublished doctoral dissertation]. Purdue University.

Fuerth, Leon, and Evan M.H. Faber. (2012). *Anticipatory Governance Practical Upgrades: Equipping the Executive Branch to Cope with Increasing Speed and Complexity of Major Challenges.* National Defense University, Center for Technology & National Security Policy.

Gordon, Milton, M. (1964). *Assimilation in American Life: The Role of Race Religion and National Origins.* Oxford University Press.

Gordon, Theodore, and Yair Sharan. (2017). "The Threat of Amplified Terrorism." Presented at the workshop "Forecasting in the Social Sciences," National Defense University, Washington, DC, July 26, 1–9.

Gotev, Georgi. (2020, April 5). "5G Coronavirus Conspiracy Theory is Dangerous Fake Nonsense, UK Says." *EurActiv.com.* Retrieved from https://advance-lexis-com.proxy.lib.wayne.edu/api/document?collection=news&id=urn:contentItem:5Y-KJ-91C1-JCF9-40KV-00000-00&context=1516831.

Gurr, Ted Robert, and Barbara Harff. (1984). *Ethnic Conflict in World Politics.* Westview Press.

Gurr, Ted Robert. (1988). "Some Characteristics of Political Terrorism in the 1960's." In Michael Stohl (Ed.), *The Politics of Terrorism, Revised and Expanded.* Marcel Dekker.

Gurr, Ted Robert. (1989). "Political Terrorism: Historical Antecedents and Contemporary Trends." In Ted Robert Gurr (Ed.), *Protest, Rebellion, Reform, Vol. 2 of Violence in America.* Sage Publications.

Harris, Rosemary. (1989). "Anthropological Views on 'Violence' in Northern Ireland." In Yonah Alexander and Alan O'Day (Eds.), *Ireland's Terrorist Trauma.* St. Martin's Press.

Henry, Nicholas. (2013). *Public Administration and Public Affairs Edition No. 12.* Pearson Education, Inc.

Im, Eric Insoon, Jon Cauley, and Todd Sandler. (1987). "Cycles and Substitutions in Terrorist Activities: A Spectral Approach." *Kyklos. 40,* 238–255.

Jacobs, Andrew. (2020, September 22). "Despite Claims, Trump Rarely Uses Wartime Law in Battle Against COVID." *New York Times.* Retrieved from https://advance-lexis-com.proxy.lib.wayne.edu/api/document?collection=news&id=urn:contentItem:60WV-5J01-JBG3-6103-00000-00&context=1516831.

Jervis, Robert. (1978). "Cooperation under the Security Dilemma." *World Politics. 30*(2), 167–214.

Kaplan, Robert D. (2000). "The Coming Anarchy." In Patrick O'Meara, Howard D. Mehlinger, Matthew Krain, and Roxana Ma Newman (Eds.), *Globalization and Challenges of A New Century: A Reader.* Indiana University Press, 34–60.

Lasswell, Harold D. (1935). *World Politics and Personal Insecurity.* McGraw Hill.

Lasswell, Harold D. (1978). "Terrorism and the Political Process." *Terrorism: An International Journal. 1*(3/4), 255–263.

Lawson, Fred. (2016). "International Relations Theory and the Middle East." In Louise Fawcett (Ed.), *International Relations in the Middle East – Fourth Edition*. Oxford University Press, 21–38.

Long, David E. (1990). *The Anatomy of Terrorism*. Free Press.

Makarenko, Tamara. (2004). "The Crime-Terror Continuum: Tracing the Interplay Between Transnational Organized Crime and Terrorism." *Global Crime*. 6(1), 129–145.

Nef, Jorge. (1978). "Some Thoughts on Contemporary Terrorism: Domestic and International Perspectives." In John Carson (Ed.), *Terrorism in Theory and Practice: Proceedings of a Colloquium*. Atlantic Council of Canada.

Nye, Joseph S., Jr. (1999). *Understanding International Conflicts: An Introduction to Theory and History – Second Edition*. HarperCollins College Publishers.

Olorunnipa, Toluse, and Cleve R. Wootson, Jr. (2020, September 30). "President Is Asked but Refuses to Condemn White Supremacists." *The Washington Post*. A-1, A-10.

Pitigala, Nihal. (2021). "The Impact of Trade and Economic Contagion on Developing and Emerging Markets." In Rohan Gunaratna and Mohd Mizan Mohammad Aslam (Eds.), *COVID-19: A Global Security Threat*. Amsterdam University Press.

Ronis, Sheila R. (2007). *Timelines into the Future: Strategic Visioning Methods for Government, Business and Other Organizations*. Hamilton Books.

Ross, Jeffrey Ian, and Ted Robert Gurr. (1989). "Why Terrorism Subsides: A Comparative Study of Canada and the United States." *Comparative Politics*. 21(4), 405–426.

Roth, A. (2020, April 6). "Bad News: Radiation 16 times above normal after forest fire near Chernobyl." *The Guardian*. http://www.the guardian.com/environment/2020/apr/06/bad-news-radiation-spikes-16- times-above-normal-after-forest-fire-near-chernobyl?fbclid=IwAR0TKjvaBPXPV7U5ijU0c3Xc93W9v1zDBZom5i_HkD4UwkRanTapRiE3UaU.

Shelley, Louise I. (2013). "Money Laundering into Real-Estate." In Michael Miklaucic and Jacqueline Brewer (Eds.), *Convergence: Illicit Networks and National Security in An Age of Globalization*. National Defense University Press, 131–146.

Thaler, David E., Ryan Andrew Brown, Gabriella C. Gonzalez, Blake W. Mobley, and Parisa Rashan. (2013). "Improving the U.S. Military's Understanding of Unstable Environments Vulnerable to Violent Extremist Groups Insights from Social Science." RAND Corporation, iii–96. https://www.rand.org/pubs/research_reports/RR298.html.

Theen, Rolf H.W., and Frank L. Wilson. (1986). *Comparative Politics an introduction to Six Countries*, Prentice-Hall.

Timberg, Craig, and Isaac Stanley-Becker. (2020, October 9). "Alleged Whitmer Kidnapping Plot Was Foreshadowed on Social Media." *The Washington Post*. A-22.

Waltz, Kenneth N. (1959). *Man, the State and War: A Theoretical Analysis*. Columbia University Press, 10–11.

Waltz, Kenneth N. (1973). "The Meaning of Anarchy." In Robert J. Art and Robert Jervis (Eds.), *International Politics: Anarchy, Force Imperialism*. Little, Brown and Company, 10–20.

Williams, Phil. (2013). "Lawlessness and Disorder: An Emerging Paradigm for the 21st Century." In Michael Miklaucic and Jacqueline Brewer (Eds.), *Convergence: Illicit Networks and National Security in An Age of Globalization*. National Defense University Press, 15–36.

Wilson, Frank L. (1990). *European Politics Today: The Democratic Experience*. Prentice-Hall.

Zapotosky, Matt, Devlin Barrett, and Abigail Hauslohner. (2020, October 9). "13 Charged in Plot to Seize Mich. Governor." *The Washington Post*. A-1, A-14.

Index

For Product Safety Concerns and Information please contact our EU
representative GPSR@taylorandfrancis.com
Taylor & Francis Verlag GmbH, Kaufingerstraße 24, 80331 München, Germany

www.ingramcontent.com/pod-product-compliance
Lightning Source LLC
Chambersburg PA
CBHW060258220326
41598CB00027B/4156

*9 7 8 1 0 3 2 0 5 4 0 6 3 *